Type 2 Diabetes Cookbook Beginner's Quick & Easy Recipes for Delicious Diabetes Diets

300 Healthy

<u>Snacks</u>

for

Diabetic Wellness in 30 minutes or Less

By

Lily Anders

Copyright Page

Ace East Publishing LLC
1401 21st Street
Suite R
Sacramento, CA 95811

ISBN: **978-1-963939-84-2**

First Edition

ACE EAST
PUBLISHING

Disclaimer Page

This cookbook is crafted to offer insightful information and recipes for those interested in managing Type 2 Diabetes through dietary choices. It is important to recognize that the authors and the publisher are not healthcare professionals. The suggestions and recipes contained within this book are not meant to replace professional medical advice, diagnoses, or treatments. Should you have any healthcare-related questions or concerns, particularly relating to Type 2 Diabetes management, we strongly advise consulting with your doctor or a qualified healthcare provider.

The culinary experiences, and recommendations shared in this book stem from extensive research and the personal journey of exploring dietary approaches to Type 2 Diabetes management. These narratives and suggestions are intended for educational and motivational purposes only, aiming to enhance understanding and inspire positive lifestyle changes, not to serve as direct medical or nutritional prescriptions.

The author(s) and publisher expressly disclaim any liability for any adverse effects arising directly or indirectly from the use and application of the information contained in this cookbook. Moreover, given the specificity and medical relevance of the content, certain topics and dietary advice may not be suitable for all readers. It is advisable for caregivers and adults to review the content before sharing with minors or individuals with particular sensitivities or health concerns.

In cases of medical emergencies or for immediate assistance with health issues, please reach out to a trusted healthcare professional or dial the emergency services number available in your locality.

The Entire Type 2 Diabetes Cookbook Series

Dive into a culinary revolution with the ***"Type 2 Diabetes Cookbook Series: Beginner's Quick & Easy Recipes for Delicious Diabetes Diets – 300 Health-Boosting Savory Meals for Diabetic Wellness in 30 Minutes or Less."***

Spread across six essential volumes – Breakfast, Lunch, Dinner, Desserts, Snacks, and Sauces, Dips, & Dressings – this series is your passport to a world where managing Type 2 Diabetes meets delicious innovation.

Each book is a treasure trove of hundreds of recipes, marrying the precision of nutritional science with the flair of culinary art. Designed for those on a diabetic diet, these recipes promise to transform your meals from bland to blissful without sacrificing flavor or health. Every dish, from energizing breakfasts to indulgent desserts, comes alive through vivid, full-color photographs, accompanied by foolproof instructions, cooking times, detailed ingredient lists, serving suggestions, and handy conversion charts.

But the journey doesn't end with tantalizing meals. These cookbooks are gateways to mastering diabetes management, offering insights into blood sugar balance, insulin functionality, and the art of carb counting. They stand as pillars of empowerment and knowledge, guiding you through the culinary and health aspects of diabetes with ease and enjoyment.

Embrace these cookbooks as more than mere collections of recipes; see them as companions in your journey toward diabetic wellness, bringing confidence, pleasure, and a burst of flavors into your daily life. Step into a world where managing diabetes is synonymous with culinary discovery and dietary joy. Welcome to your new kitchen adventure!

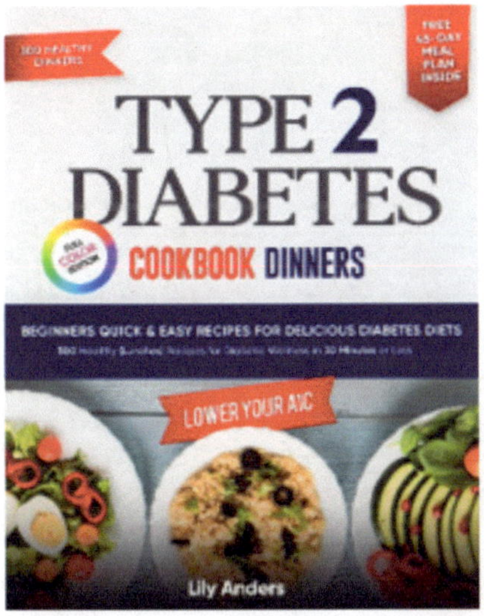
TYPE 2
DIABETES
COOKBOOK DINNERS
BEGINNERS QUICK & EASY RECIPES FOR DELICIOUS DIABETES DIETS
LOWER YOUR A1C
Lily Anders

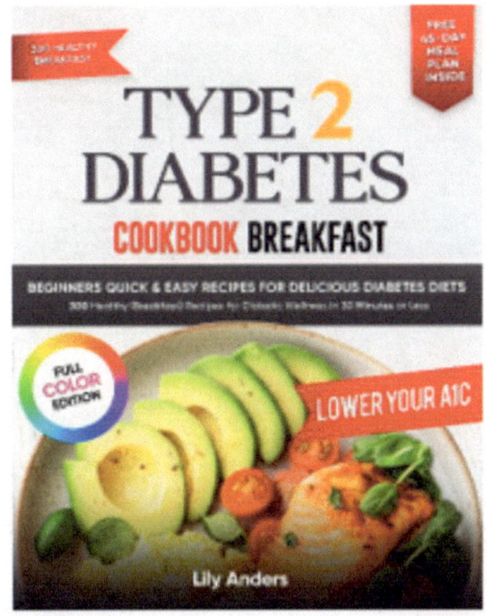
TYPE 2
DIABETES
COOKBOOK BREAKFAST
BEGINNERS QUICK & EASY RECIPES FOR DELICIOUS DIABETES DIETS
FULL COLOR EDITION
LOWER YOUR A1C
Lily Anders

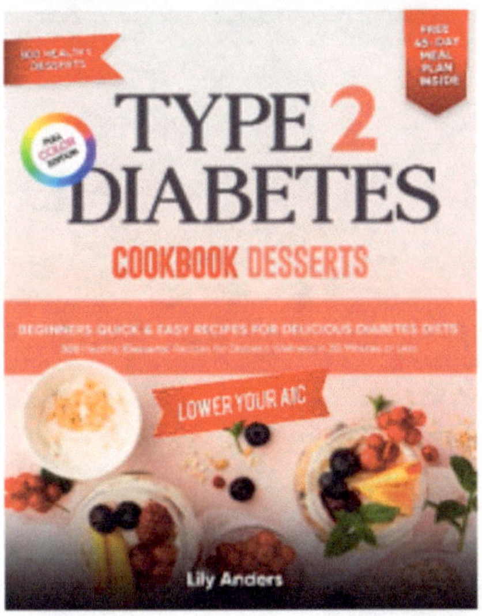
TYPE 2
DIABETES
COOKBOOK DESSERTS
LOWER YOUR A1C
Lily Anders

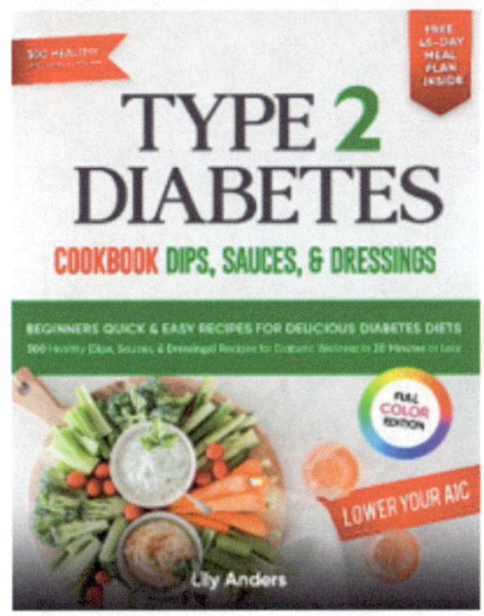
TYPE 2
DIABETES
COOKBOOK DIPS, SAUCES, & DRESSINGS
BEGINNERS QUICK & EASY RECIPES FOR DELICIOUS DIABETES DIETS
LOWER YOUR A1C
Lily Anders

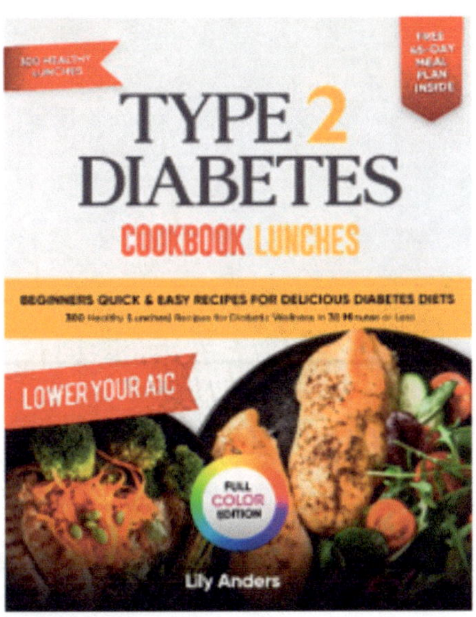
TYPE 2
DIABETES
COOKBOOK LUNCHES
BEGINNERS QUICK & EASY RECIPES FOR DELICIOUS DIABETES DIETS
LOWER YOUR A1C
Lily Anders

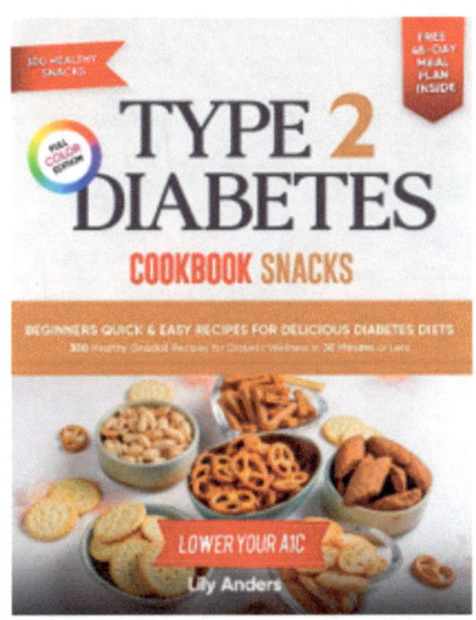
TYPE 2
DIABETES
COOKBOOK SNACKS
BEGINNERS QUICK & EASY RECIPES FOR DELICIOUS DIABETES DIETS
LOWER YOUR A1C
Lily Anders

Here's My Promise to You!

To jumpstart your journey toward healthier eating, here is the remaining

Listing of 200 Delicious & Diabetes-Friendly Snack Recipes!

That's right—you now have access to a treasure trove of 200 additional diabetic recipes designed to help you enjoy flavorful, balanced meals while managing your blood sugar with confidence. These Snack recipes will inspire you to create satisfying, nutritious meals with ease.

☞ CLICK THE LINK OR SCAN THE QR CODE TO DOWNLOAD YOUR FREE RECIPE COLLECTION!

Enjoy, and Happy Cooking!

The journey to better health starts with the right food choices, and this cookbook and it is here to support you every step of the way.

Thank you for trusting this guide, and here's to a flavorful, balanced, and empowered approach to managing Type 2 Diabetes!

You've got this! □□✨

<<Click here to access your 45 day meal plan>>

https://acrobat.adobe.com/id/urn:aaid:sc:VA6C2:448a7fa7-ffcd-4919-9d29-1c8e6bee62e9

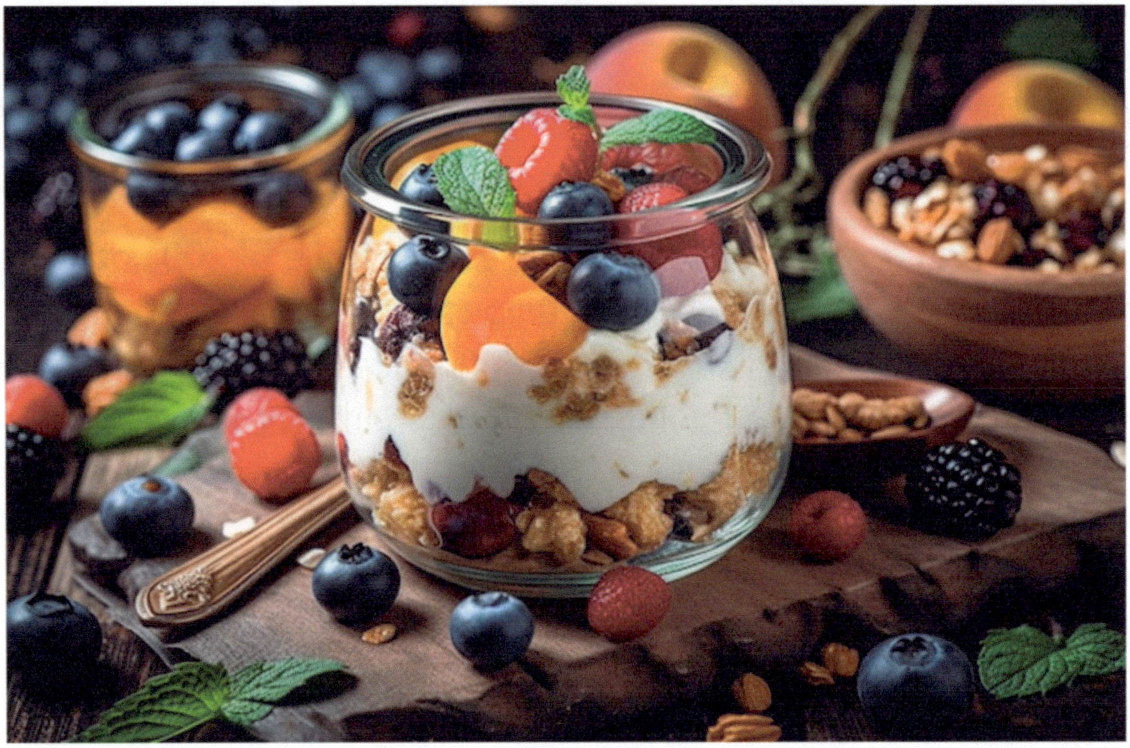

1. Greek Yogurt Parfait with Berries and Almonds

Prep.Time:	Cook Time:	Serving:	Beverage pairing:
5 min	0 min	1	Herbal Tea

Ingredients:

- 1 cup Greek yogurt (low-fat or non-fat)
- 1/2 cup mixed berries (such as strawberries, blueberries, raspberries)
- 1 tablespoon sliced almonds

Preparation:

1. In a serving glass or bowl, layer the Greek yogurt.
2. Top with mixed berries.
3. Sprinkle sliced almonds on top.

Nutrient Facts (per serving):

- Calories: Approximately 200 per serving
- Carbohydrates: 20g
- Fat: 8g
- Protein: 15g

Table of Contents

INTRODUCTION

Supporting Your Day Between Meals

For many people managing Type 2 Diabetes, snacks create the most uncertainty. Hunger appears between meals, energy dips unexpectedly, and the right choice can feel unclear. Snacking is often associated with guilt, fear, or frustration, especially when blood sugar stability is a concern.

Yet snacks play an important role in daily balance.

When chosen thoughtfully, snacks help regulate hunger, prevent energy crashes, and support consistent blood sugar levels throughout the day. When ignored or approached without structure, they can lead to overeating later, impulsive choices, or unnecessary stress.

This book was written to remove that uncertainty.

The Type 2 Diabetes Cookbook: Snacks focuses on balanced, diabetes-conscious snacks designed to support your body between meals. These recipes are practical, portion-aware, and easy to incorporate into everyday life, whether you are at home, at work, or on the go.

Snacks are not meant to replace meals. They are meant to support them. A well-chosen snack can help bridge long gaps between meals, stabilize energy, and reduce the temptation to overeat later in the day.

The good news is that diabetes-friendly snacks do not need to be bland, restrictive, or complicated.

Inside this book, you will find snack options that are both satisfying and supportive, emphasizing protein, fiber, and healthy fats to help maintain balance. Each recipe is designed to be simple to prepare and easy to enjoy without guilt.

This cookbook is not about constant monitoring or strict rules. It is about building confidence around eating between meals and understanding how snacks fit into your overall routine.

You do not need to avoid snacking. You need a plan that works.

Welcome to a calmer, more confident approach to snacking with Type 2 Diabetes.

Chapter 1

Understanding Type 2 Diabetes Between Meals

Between meals is often where the day feels hardest to manage. Hunger appears unexpectedly, energy dips, and decisions must be made quickly. For many people managing Type 2 Diabetes, these moments can trigger anxiety, guilt, or confusion about what to eat next.

Type 2 Diabetes influences how the body uses insulin, the hormone that helps move glucose from the bloodstream into the cells for energy. When insulin does not work as efficiently as it should, glucose can remain in the blood longer than intended. This process is ongoing throughout the day, not only during main meals. How you handle the gaps between meals matters just as much as what you choose at breakfast, lunch, or dinner.

Snacks are not a sign of weakness or failure. They are an opportunity to support balance.

Why Between-Meal Moments Are Critical

After a meal, blood sugar rises and then gradually falls. If the next meal is far away, hunger or low energy can build. When hunger becomes intense, it is easier to reach for quick options that may be high in refined carbohydrates or added sugar, leading to sharp rises and falls in blood sugar.

These swings can create a cycle of fatigue, cravings, or overeating. Over time, this pattern may make diabetes management feel more difficult and less predictable.

When snacks are chosen thoughtfully, they help bridge the gap between meals. They reduce sudden hunger, support steadier energy, and decrease the chance of impulsive choices later in the day.

Practical Role of Snacks

The goal is not to eat constantly. The goal is to use snacks in a way that supports your overall routine. A well-chosen snack can keep you comfortable, focused, and in control until the next meal.

Healthy snacking can fit into a daily meal pattern, and some guidance suggests eating at regular times with a couple of hours between meals to give blood sugar time to settle. This creates a rhythm that can reduce confusion and support consistency.

What Makes a Supportive Snack

Supportive snacks provide a balance of nutrients rather than relying on carbohydrates alone. Protein, healthy fats, and fiber help slow digestion, add satisfaction, and promote steadier blood sugar levels.

Some practical combinations suggested by a reputable diabetes resource include fruit with cheese or nuts, hummus or guacamole with vegetables, and nut butter with fruit or vegetables. These choices illustrate how protein and healthy fats can enhance carbohydrate-containing foods, making snacks both more satisfying and more supportive of balance.

Removing Fear Around Snacking

Fear often comes from uncertainty. If snacks feel risky or confusing, it is natural to avoid them altogether or to choose something impulsive. This book aims to remove the fear by providing clear, practical options that fit real life.

You will not need to follow strict rules or monitor every bite. Instead, you will learn patterns that consistently support balance between meals, helping you feel more confident and less reactive during the day.

Building Confidence Through Routine

As you begin to use supportive snacks, you will notice patterns. Some options keep you full longer, some are easier to prepare, and some fit better with your schedule. This experience builds confidence, and over time, choosing snacks becomes intuitive.

When snacks are practical, balanced, and enjoyable, they become a useful tool, not a source of stress.

In the next chapter, we will explore how hunger and energy behave between meals, and why certain snack combinations help prevent sudden drops or cravings later in the day.

Chapter 2

Hunger, Energy, and the Between-Meal Window

Hunger between meals is not a failure of discipline. It is a signal. For individuals managing Type 2 Diabetes, understanding what that signal means can help prevent energy dips, cravings, and frustration throughout the day.

Between meals, blood sugar levels naturally begin to fall as the body uses glucose for energy. When this decline is gradual, hunger remains manageable. When it happens quickly, hunger can feel sudden and intense, often accompanied by fatigue or difficulty concentrating.

Why Energy Drops Between Meals

Energy drops commonly occur when previous meals were unbalanced or when too much time passes without nourishment. Meals that rely heavily on refined carbohydrates can cause blood sugar levels to rise quickly and then fall sharply. This rapid change often leads to a strong desire for quick energy.

In contrast, meals that include protein, fiber, and healthy fats support a slower release of glucose. This helps extend energy and delay hunger.

Recognizing this pattern makes it easier to plan snacks that support balance rather than react to discomfort.

The Between-Meal Window Explained

The between-meal window refers to the period after digestion of a meal has begun but before the next meal is consumed. During this time, the body relies on stored energy and gradual glucose release.

For individuals with Type 2 Diabetes, this window can be unpredictable. Stress, physical activity, sleep, and timing of meals all influence how hunger and energy are experienced.

Well-timed snacks can help smooth this window, preventing sharp declines in energy and reducing the urge to overeat at the next meal.

Timing Snacks for Stability

Snacks are most helpful when they are planned rather than reactive. Waiting until hunger becomes intense often leads to choices that prioritize speed over balance.

A small, balanced snack eaten before hunger becomes overwhelming can help maintain steady energy and improve focus. This approach supports better blood sugar regulation and reduces stress around food.

Spacing meals and snacks consistently throughout the day helps create predictability and routine.

Choosing Snacks That Support Energy

Snacks designed to support energy should include more than carbohydrates alone. Protein slows digestion and promotes fullness, while healthy fats contribute to satisfaction. Fiber further moderates blood sugar response.

This combination helps extend energy and reduce the likelihood of cravings. Snacks that are balanced tend to feel more satisfying, even when portions are modest.

Responding to Hunger Without Guilt

Hunger is a natural part of daily life. Responding to it thoughtfully supports long-term consistency and confidence.

This book encourages listening to hunger cues and using snacks as a tool rather than viewing them as a problem. When snacks are planned and balanced, they become part of a supportive routine.

In the next chapter, we will focus on carbohydrates in snacks, how to include them without excess, and how pairing choices can make a meaningful difference between meals.

Chapter 3

Carbohydrates in Snacks Without Spikes

Carbohydrates are often the first nutrient people question when choosing a snack. Many common snack foods are carbohydrate-heavy and quick to digest, which can lead to sharp rises and falls in blood sugar. This can make snacking feel risky for individuals managing Type 2 Diabetes.

The goal with snacks is not to avoid carbohydrates entirely. It is to include them in ways that support steady energy and predictable blood sugar responses.

Why Snack Carbohydrates Behave Differently

Snacks are typically smaller than meals, yet they can still have a significant impact on blood sugar. When carbohydrates are eaten alone, especially refined carbohydrates, glucose can enter the bloodstream quickly. Without other nutrients to slow digestion, blood sugar levels may spike and then drop soon after.

These rapid changes often lead to renewed hunger or cravings shortly after snacking, creating a cycle that feels difficult to manage.

Understanding how carbohydrates behave in snack-sized portions helps remove fear and supports better choices.

Choosing Carbohydrates That Digest Slowly

Carbohydrates that contain fiber are digested more slowly and create a gentler blood sugar response. Fruits, vegetables, whole grains, and legumes provide carbohydrates that are more supportive when used thoughtfully.

For example, berries, apples, and pears offer fiber along with natural sweetness. Whole-grain crackers or small portions of whole grains can also fit into balanced snacks when paired appropriately.

The quality of carbohydrates matters just as much as the quantity.

Pairing to Prevent Spikes

One of the most effective ways to include carbohydrates in snacks is through pairing. Protein and healthy fats slow digestion and help prevent rapid blood sugar rises.

A snack that includes carbohydrates along with protein or fat often feels more satisfying and supports longer-lasting energy. This combination reduces the likelihood of spikes and crashes between meals.

Pairing does not need to be complicated. Simple combinations can make a meaningful difference.

Portion Awareness for Snack Balance

Even supportive carbohydrates can create challenges when portions are larger than needed. Snack portions should feel satisfying without feeling heavy.

Smaller portions paired with protein or fat often provide better results than larger carbohydrate-only snacks. This approach allows carbohydrates to remain part of snacking without overwhelming the body.

Building Confidence Through Practice

As you experiment with different snack combinations, patterns will begin to emerge. Some snacks will keep you energized longer, while others may lead to quicker hunger.

This experience builds confidence and helps you learn what works best for your body. Snacking becomes less about fear and more about intention.

In the next chapter, we will focus on smart snack shopping, helping you choose ingredients and options that make balanced snacking easier throughout the day.

Chapter 4

Smart Snack Shopping

Smart snack shopping removes much of the stress around eating between meals. When supportive snack options are readily available, it becomes easier to respond to hunger thoughtfully rather than reactively. For individuals managing Type 2 Diabetes, this preparation helps maintain steady energy and blood sugar balance throughout the day.

Snack shopping does not require specialty stores or complicated products. It requires intention and familiarity with dependable options.

Shopping With Between-Meal Needs in Mind

Snacks are meant to bridge the gap between meals, not replace them. When shopping, it helps to choose foods that are easy to portion, quick to access, and supportive of balance.

Protein-rich items such as nuts, seeds, yogurt, cheese, eggs, and legumes form a strong foundation for snacking. These foods promote fullness and slow digestion, helping prevent sudden hunger or energy drops.

Vegetables and fruits add fiber and nutrients, making them valuable snack components. Fresh, frozen, or pre-cut options all work well, depending on convenience and preference.

Navigating Packaged Snack Foods

Packaged snacks are widely available, but many are high in refined carbohydrates, added sugars, or oversized portions. Snack bars, crackers, and baked goods often appear convenient yet may cause blood sugar fluctuations.

When choosing packaged snacks, focus on simple ingredient lists and balanced nutrition. Look for options that include protein or fiber rather than relying solely on carbohydrates.

Single-serving packages can be helpful for portion awareness, especially when snacking away from home.

Choosing Snacks for Portability

Snacks are often eaten on the go, at work, or between commitments. Choosing portable options supports consistency and reduces the temptation to skip snacks or make impulsive choices.

Shelf-stable items such as nuts, seeds, nut butters, and whole-grain crackers can be paired easily with fruits or vegetables. Refrigerated options, when packed properly, offer additional variety.

Planning for portability helps ensure that balanced snacks are available when hunger appears.

Creating a Reliable Snack List

Having a short list of reliable snack options simplifies shopping and decision-making. This list may include a few protein sources, fiber-rich produce, and healthy fats that can be combined in different ways.

Rotating familiar snacks reduces boredom while maintaining structure. This approach supports consistency without overwhelming choice.

Making Snack Shopping Sustainable

Effective snack shopping supports long-term habits. As you become familiar with dependable options, shopping becomes faster and more intuitive.

When your environment supports balanced snacking, hunger between meals becomes easier to manage and less stressful.

In the next chapter, we will explore simple preparation strategies that make snacks easy to assemble and enjoy, even on the busiest days.

Chapter 5

Prep Strategies for Easy Snacking

Snacks are most effective when they are easy to access and simple to prepare. When hunger appears suddenly, the path of least resistance often determines what is eaten. For individuals managing Type 2 Diabetes, having prepared snack options available helps prevent rushed choices that may disrupt blood sugar balance.

Preparation does not need to be time-consuming. Small, intentional steps can make a significant difference.

Preparing Snacks Ahead of Time

Preparing snacks in advance removes much of the effort from between-meal decisions. Washing and portioning fruits and vegetables, dividing nuts into small containers, or preparing yogurt and cottage cheese servings ahead of time help make balanced snacks immediately available.

Hard-boiled eggs, cut vegetables, and pre-portioned cheese are examples of snacks that can be prepared once and enjoyed over several days. These options support protein intake and help extend energy between meals.

Even minimal preparation can improve consistency.

Building Snack Kits

Snack kits are combinations of two or three simple items that work well together. Creating a few reliable snack combinations reduces decision fatigue and makes snacking feel intentional rather than reactive.

For example, pairing fruit with a protein source or vegetables with a healthy fat creates balance. Keeping these items together in the refrigerator or pantry makes them easy to grab when needed.

Snack kits are especially helpful for workdays, travel, or busy schedules.

Using Portion-Friendly Containers

Portion awareness is easier when snacks are pre-portioned. Small containers or reusable bags help prevent overeating and remove the need for measuring during busy moments.

Pre-portioned snacks provide visual cues that support balance. When portions are already set, it becomes easier to eat mindfully and stop when satisfied.

This approach encourages consistency without strict rules.

Keeping Backup Options Available

Not every day allows for preparation, and that is expected. Keeping a few shelf-stable backup snacks helps ensure that balanced options are still available.

Items such as nuts, seeds, nut butter packets, and whole-grain crackers can be stored in a desk, bag, or car. These options provide support during unexpected hunger or schedule changes.

Backup snacks are not a substitute for regular meals, but they are a valuable safety net.

Creating a Supportive Snacking Routine

Consistency makes snacking easier and less stressful. Developing a loose routine, such as having a snack at similar times each day, helps regulate hunger and energy levels.

This routine does not need to be rigid. It simply provides structure that supports better decision-making.

In the next chapter, we will focus on portion awareness for snacks, helping you enjoy satisfying options without overeating or disrupting blood sugar balance.

Chapter 6

Portion Awareness for Balanced Snacking

Portion size is one of the most important factors in effective snacking. Even well-chosen snacks can disrupt blood sugar balance when portions are larger than the body needs between meals. Understanding portion awareness helps snacks remain supportive rather than overwhelming.

Portion awareness is not about restriction. It is about choosing an amount that satisfies hunger without creating discomfort or unnecessary blood sugar fluctuations.

Why Snack Portions Matter

Snacks are meant to fill the gap between meals, not replace them. When snack portions are too large, they can reduce appetite for the next meal or contribute to blood sugar spikes.

For individuals managing Type 2 Diabetes, oversized snack portions that are high in carbohydrates may lead to rapid increases in blood sugar followed by quick declines. These swings can trigger renewed hunger or fatigue.

Balanced portions help maintain steady energy and make it easier to transition smoothly to the next meal.

Recognizing Balanced Snack Portions

A balanced snack portion should feel satisfying without feeling heavy. Protein, healthy fats, and fiber help make smaller portions more effective by slowing digestion and extending fullness.

Visual cues can be helpful. A snack that fits comfortably in the hand or a small container is often sufficient. When snacks are paired thoughtfully, less is usually needed to feel satisfied.

Eating slowly and without distraction can also improve portion awareness, allowing hunger cues to guide intake.

Common Snacking Portion Challenges

Snacking often occurs while multitasking, which can make it difficult to notice fullness. Eating directly from large containers or packages increases the likelihood of overeating.

Portion challenges can also arise when snacks are used to cope with stress or boredom rather than hunger. Recognizing the difference between physical hunger and emotional cues helps guide better choices.

These challenges are common and manageable with awareness.

Adjusting Portions to Fit Your Day

Portion needs may vary depending on activity level, timing of meals, and overall energy demands. On more active days, slightly larger snack portions may feel appropriate. On less active days, smaller portions may be sufficient.

Flexibility allows snacks to support your routine without becoming rigid or stressful.

Building Confidence Through Consistency

Over time, portion awareness becomes intuitive. As you repeat balanced snack choices, your body begins to respond more predictably, and confidence grows.

The snack recipes in this book are designed with portion awareness in mind, helping remove guesswork and support balanced snacking.

In the next section, we will transition into the snack recipes, where these principles are applied through practical, satisfying options designed for real life.

Supporting Balance Between Meals

The guidance you have explored in this section is meant to simplify how you approach snacking, not add pressure or complexity. Understanding hunger cues, learning how to include carbohydrates thoughtfully, and developing practical habits around shopping, preparation, and portion awareness all serve one purpose. . . to help you navigate the spaces between meals with confidence.

Now it is time to put those principles into practice.

The snack recipes that follow are designed to support steady energy and balanced blood sugar throughout the day. Each option emphasizes simple combinations of protein, fiber, and healthy fats, helping snacks feel satisfying rather than temporary. These recipes are practical, portion-aware, and easy to incorporate into real-life routines.

You do not need to prepare every recipe or follow them in order. Choose snacks that fit your schedule, your environment, and your hunger patterns. Some days may call for something quick and portable, while others may allow for a more intentional pause. Both approaches are supported here.

As you explore the recipes, pay attention to how different snacks affect your energy, focus, and appetite. Use that awareness to guide future choices and refine what works best for you.

This section is not about constant restraint or rigid rules. It is about using snacks as a supportive tool that helps you move through the day with steadiness and ease.

Let these recipes help you stay nourished, focused, and confident between meals.

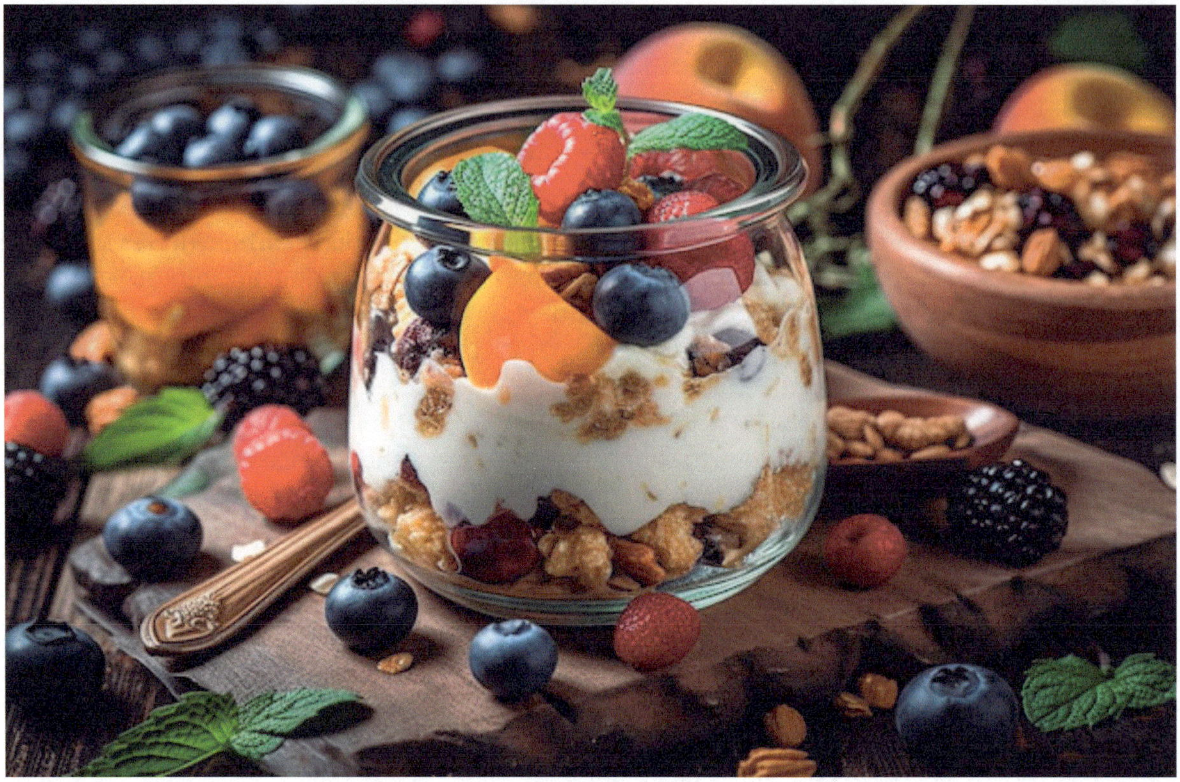

1. Greek Yogurt Parfait with Berries and Almonds

Prep.Time: 5 min	**Cook Time:** 0 min	**Serving:** 1	**Beverage pairing:** Herbal Tea

Ingredients:

- 1 cup Greek yogurt (low-fat or non-fat)
- 1/2 cup mixed berries (such as strawberries, blueberries, raspberries)
- 1 tablespoon sliced almonds

Preparation:

1. In a serving glass or bowl, layer the Greek yogurt.
2. Top with mixed berries.
3. Sprinkle sliced almonds on top.

Nutrient Facts (per serving):

- Calories: Approximately 200 per serving
- Carbohydrates: 20g
- Fat: 8g
- Protein: 15g

2. Celery Sticks with Peanut Butter

Prep.Time:	Cook Time:	Serving:	Beverage pairing:
5 min	0 min	1	Lemonade

Ingredients:

- 2 celery stalks, washed and trimmed
- 2 tablespoons peanut butter (sugar-free)

Preparation:

1. Cut the celery stalks into sticks.
2. Spread peanut butter on one side of each celery stick.

Nutrient Facts (per serving):

- Calories: Approximately 150 per serving
- Carbohydrates: 8g
- Fat: 12g
- Protein: 6g

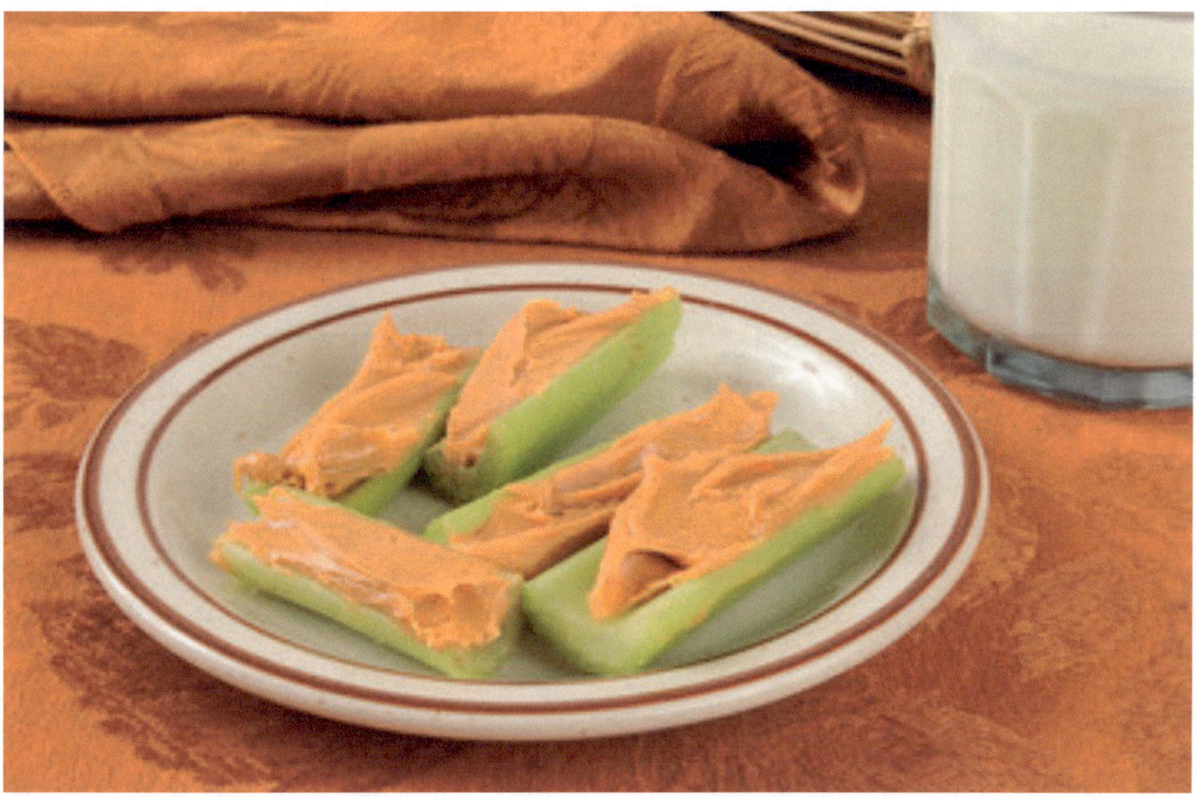

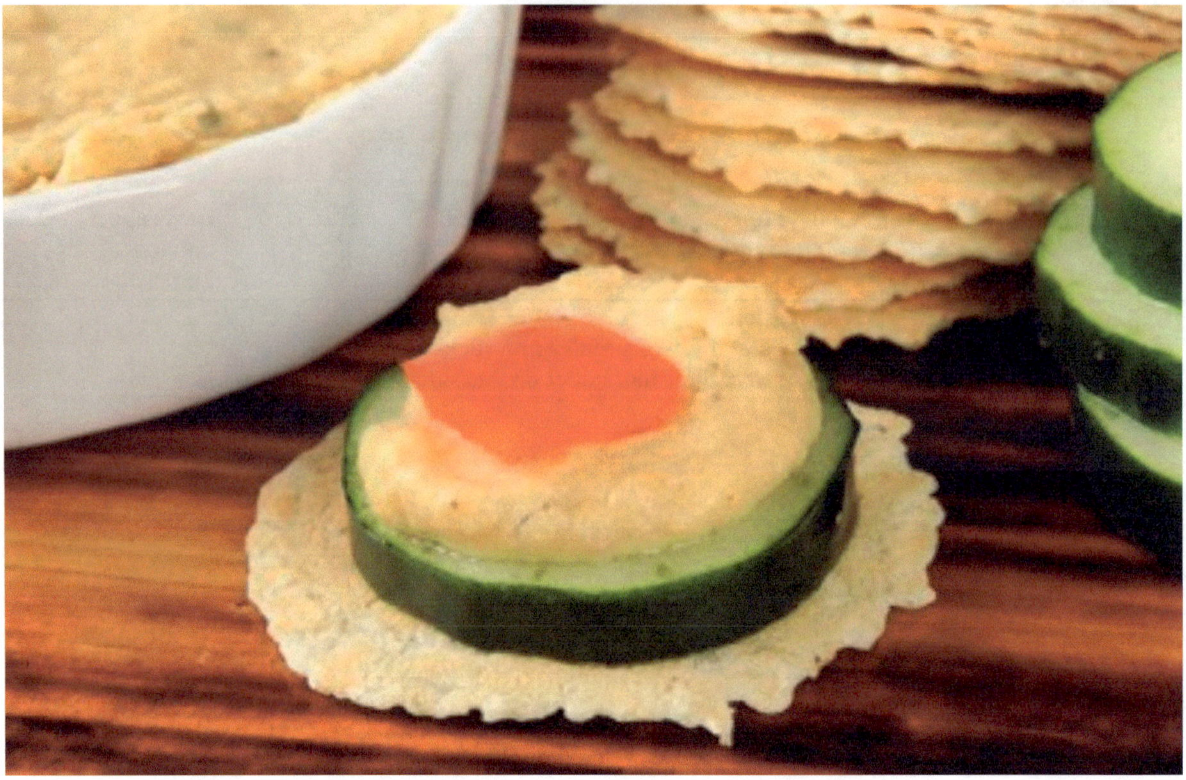

3. Cucumber Slices with Hummus

Prep.Time: 5 min	**Cook Time:** 0 min	**Serving:** 1	**Beverage pairing:** Herbal Tea

Ingredients:

- 1 medium cucumber, sliced
- 1/4 cup hummus

Preparation:

1. Wash and slice the cucumber.
2. Serve with hummus for dipping.

Nutrient Facts (per serving):

- Calories: Approximately 120 per serving
- Carbohydrates: 10g
- Fat: 7g
- Protein: 5g

4. Hard-Boiled Eggs with a Sprinkle of Salt

Prep.Time:	Cook Time:	Serving:	Beverage pairing:
3 min	15 min	1	Chamomile Tea

Ingredients:

- 2 hard-boiled eggs
- Pinch of salt

Preparation:

1. Peel the hard-boiled eggs.
2. Sprinkle with a pinch of salt.

Nutrient Facts (per serving):

- Calories: Approximately 70 per serving
- Carbohydrates: 0g
- Fat: 5g
- Protein: 6g

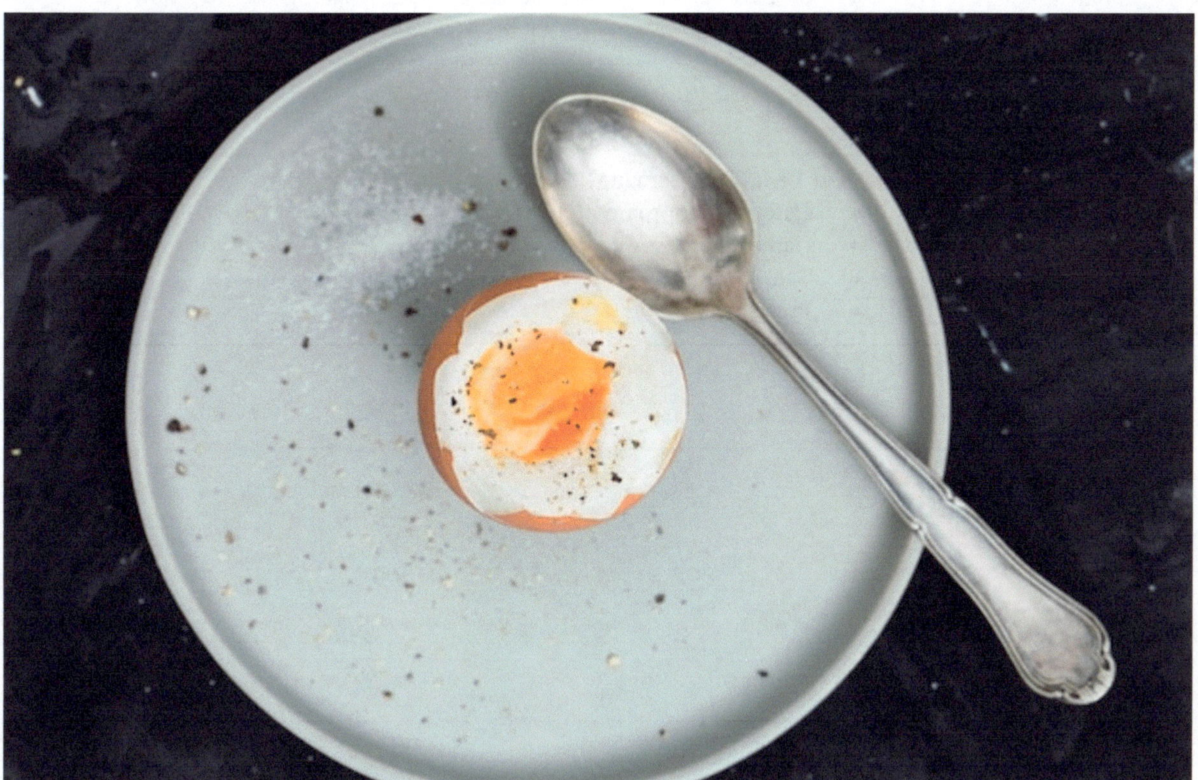

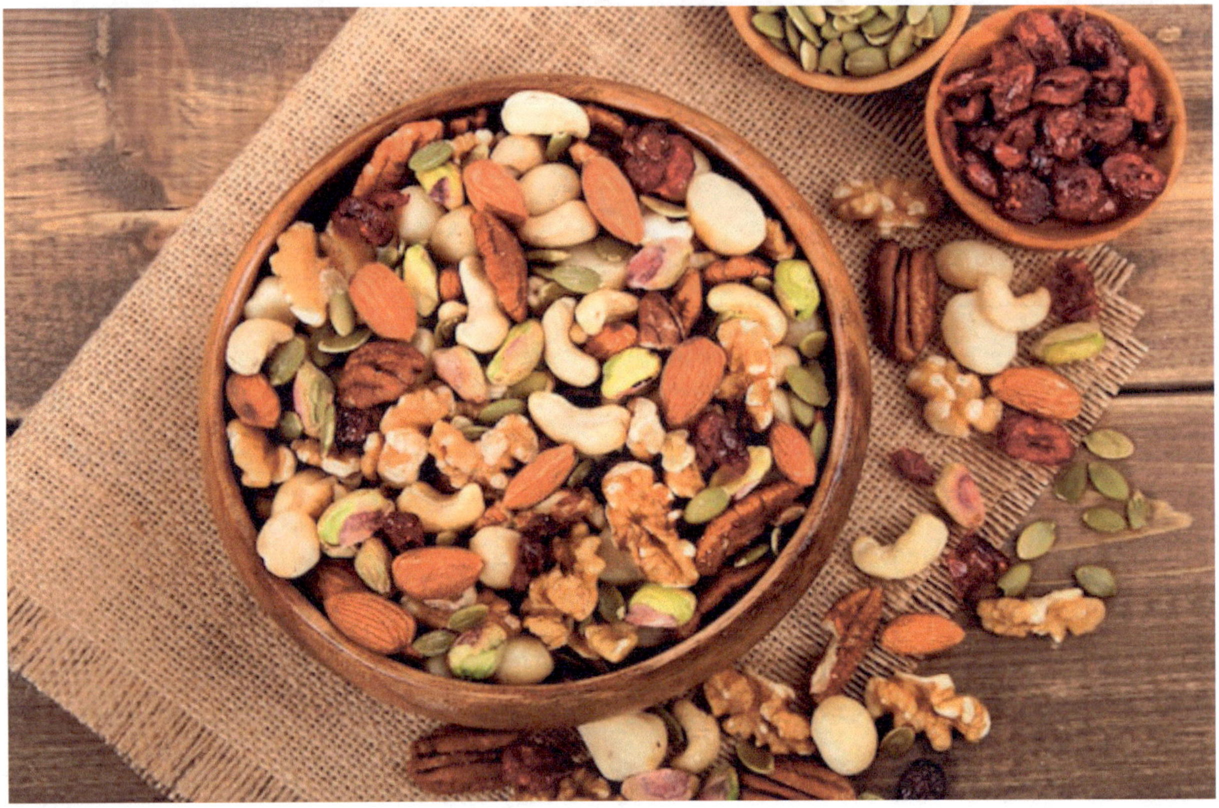

5. Mixed Nuts and Seeds Trail Mix

Prep.Time: 5 min

Cook Time: 0 min

Serving: 1

Beverage pairing: Black Coffee

Ingredients:

- 1/4 cup almonds
- 1/4 cup walnuts
- 1/4 cup pumpkin seeds
- 1/4 cup sunflower seeds
- 1/4 cup dried cranberries (sugar-free)

Preparation:

1. Mix all the nuts, seeds, and dried cranberries together in a bowl.
2. Portion into single-serving bags for convenience.

Nutrient Facts (per serving):

- Calories: Approximately 180 per serving
- Carbohydrates: 6g
- Fat: 15g
- Protein: 8g

6. Cheese Cubes and Cherry Tomatoes Skewers

Prep.Time: 5 min

Cook Time: 0 min

Serving: 1

Beverage pairing: Almond Milk

Ingredients:

- 1 ounce cheese cubes (such as cheddar or mozzarella)
- 1/2 cup cherry tomatoes
- Skewers

Preparation:

1. Thread cheese cubes and cherry tomatoes onto skewers in alternating patterns.

Nutrient Facts (per serving):

- Calories: Approximately 120 per serving
- Carbohydrates: 4g
- Fat: 8g
- Protein: 6g

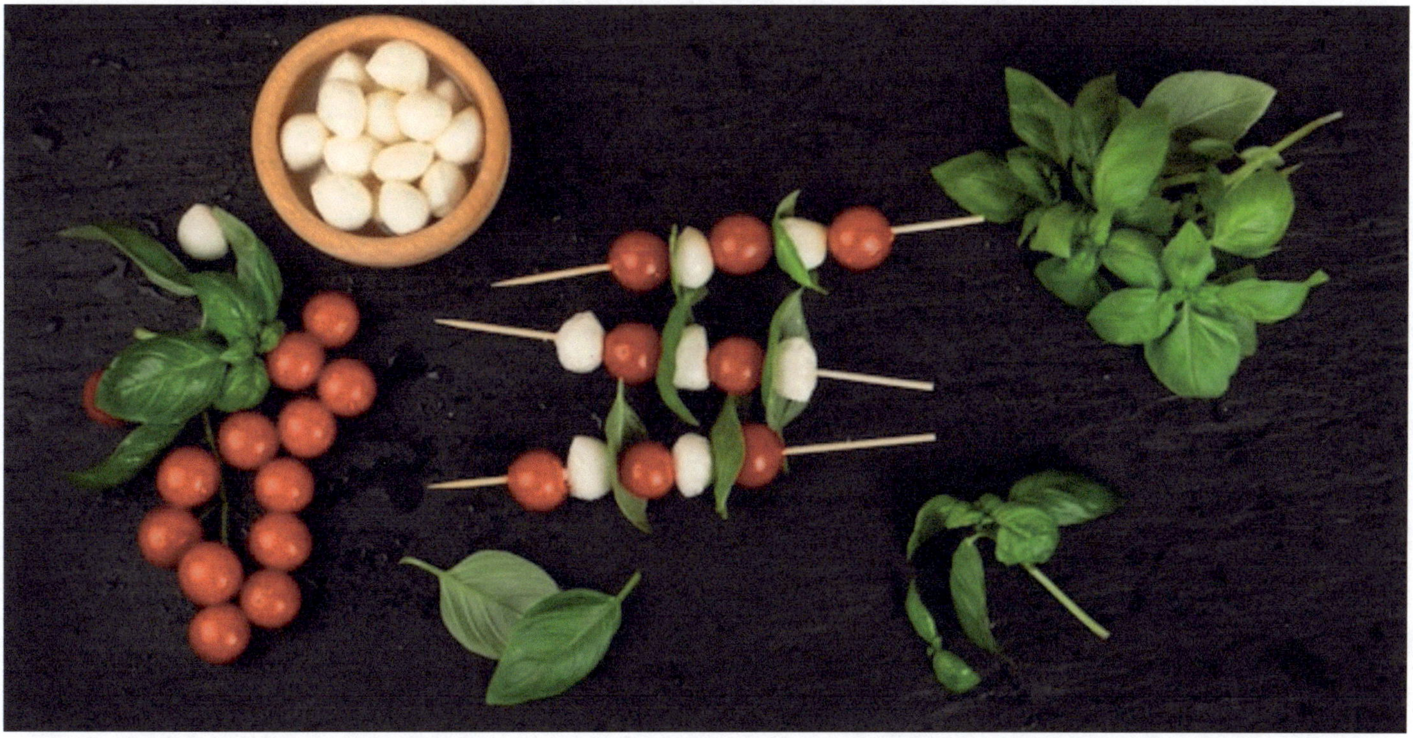

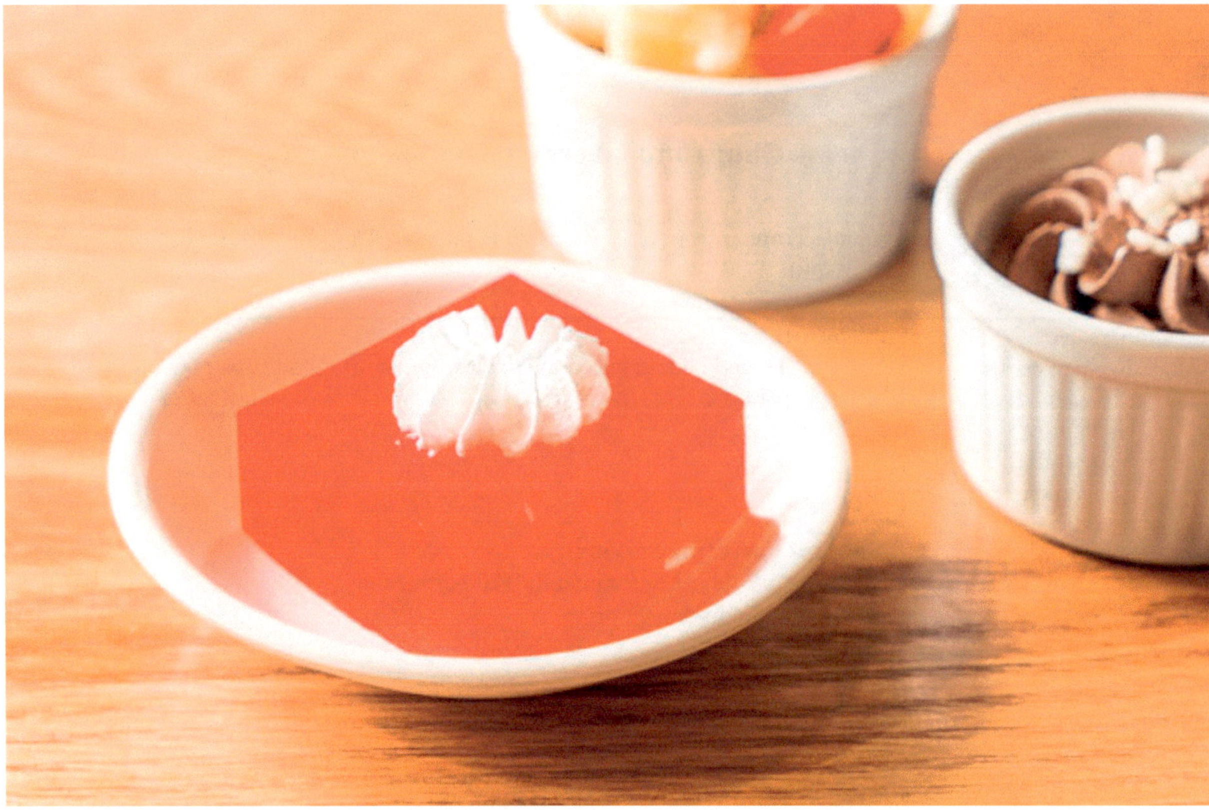

7. Sugar-Free Jello with Whipped Cream

Prep.Time:	Cook Time:	Serving:	Beverage pairing:
5 min	2-4 Hour	1	Herbal Tea

Ingredients:

- 1 sugar-free Jello cup (gelatin)
- 2 tablespoons whipped cream (sugar-free)

Preparation:

1. Prepare the sugar-free Jello according to package instructions and let it set.
2. Top with whipped cream before serving.

Nutrient Facts (per serving):

- Calories: Approximately 30 per serving
- Carbohydrates: 1g
- Fat: 2g
- Protein: 1g

8. Avocado Slices with Lemon Pepper

Prep.Time:	Cook Time:	Serving:	Beverage pairing:
5 min	0 min	1	Green Tea

Ingredients:

- 1 ripe avocado, sliced
- Lemon pepper seasoning

Preparation:

1. Slice the avocado and arrange the slices on a plate.
2. Sprinkle lemon pepper seasoning over the avocado slices.

Nutrient Facts (per serving):

- Calories: Approximately 120 per serving
- Carbohydrates: 6g
- Fat: 11g
- Protein: 2g

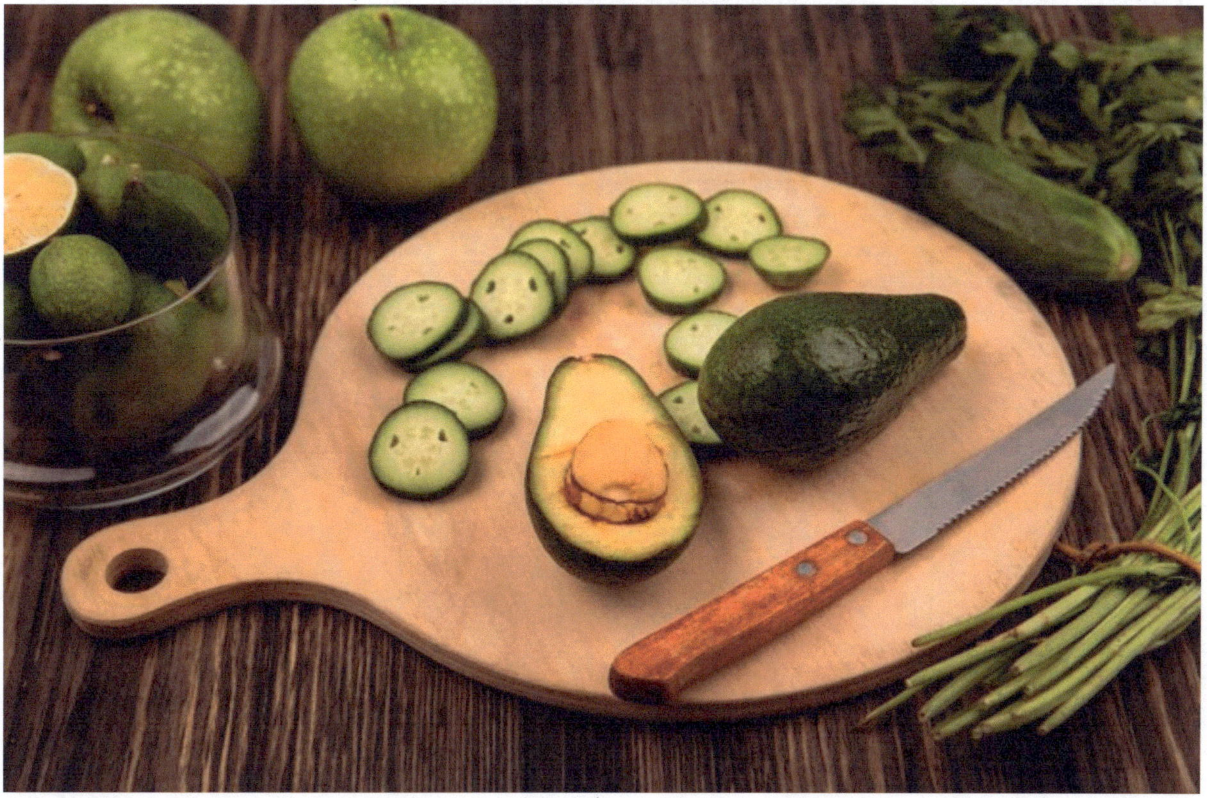

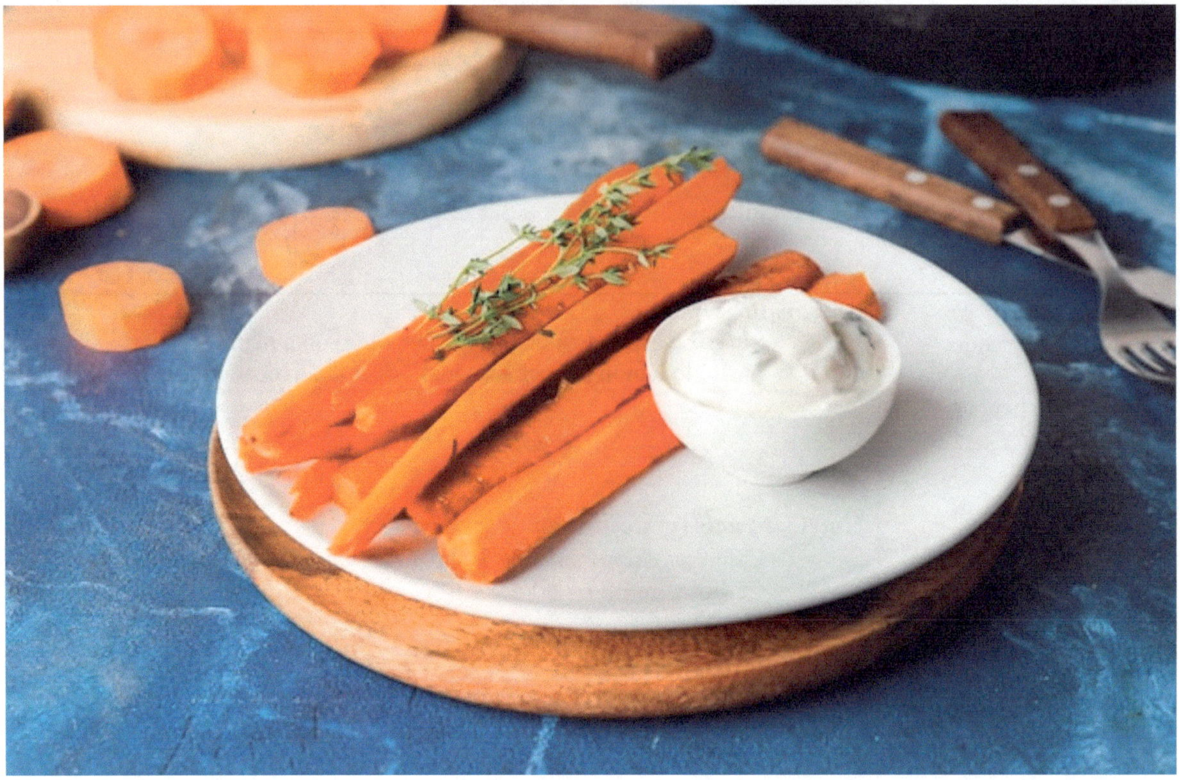

9. Carrot Sticks with Tzatziki Sauce

Prep.Time:	Cook Time:	Serving:	Beverage pairing:
5 min	0 min	1	Mint Tea

Ingredients:

- 1 large carrot, peeled and cut into sticks
- 2 tablespoons tzatziki sauce

Preparation:

1. Peel the carrot and cut it into sticks.
2. Serve with tzatziki sauce for dipping.

Nutrient Facts (per serving):

- Calories: Approximately 70 per serving
- Carbohydrates: 7g
- Fat: 4g
- Protein: 2g

10. Baked Kale Chips with Olive Oil

Prep.Time:	Cook Time:	Serving:	Beverage pairing:
0 min	10-15 min	1	Herbal Tea

Ingredients:

- 2 cups kale leaves, washed and torn into bite-sized pieces
- 1 tablespoon olive oil
- Salt to taste

Preparation:

1. Preheat the oven to 350°F (175°C).
2. In a bowl, toss the kale leaves with olive oil until coated.
3. Spread the kale leaves in a single layer on a baking sheet.
4. Sprinkle with salt.
5. Bake for 10-15 minutes until crispy.

Nutrient Facts (per serving):

- Calories: Approximately 80 per serving
- Carbohydrates: 5g
- Fat: 5g
- Protein: 3g

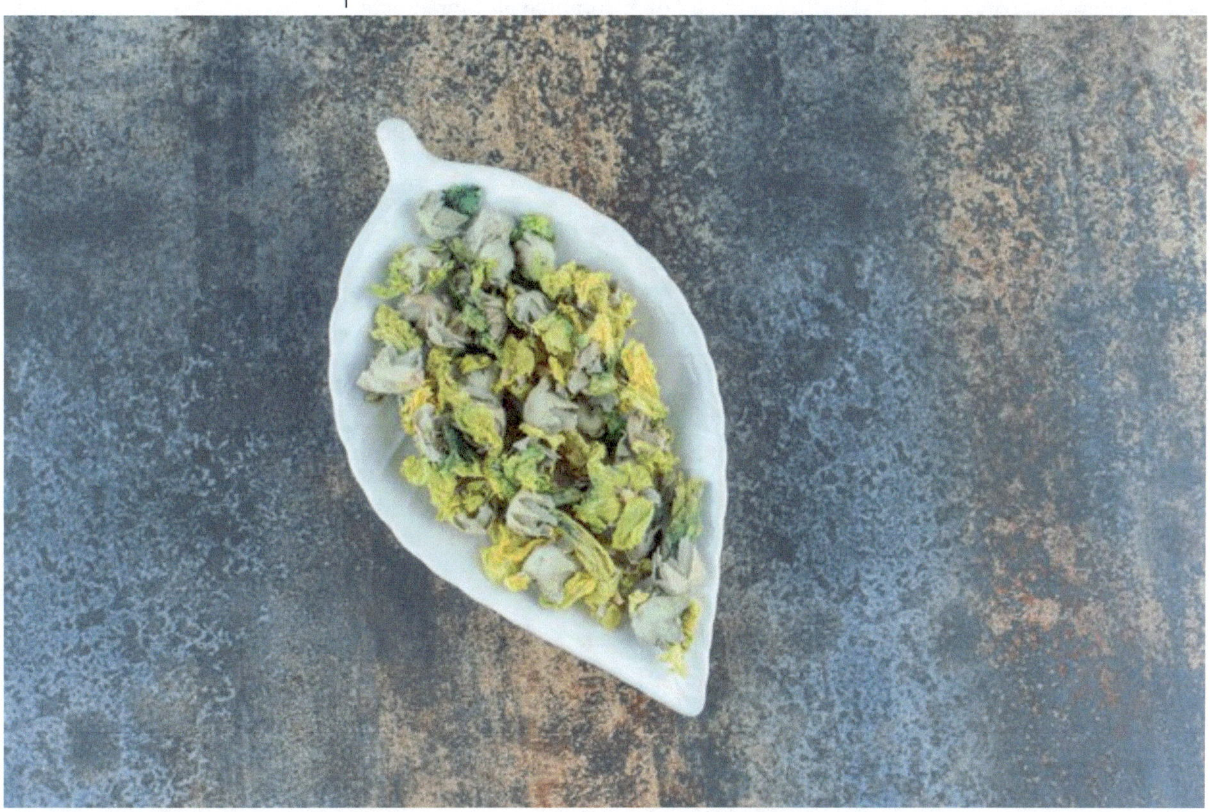

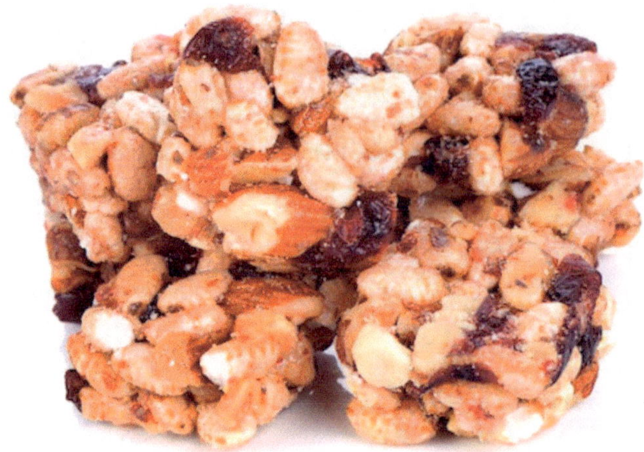

11. Cherry Almond Energy Bites

Prep.Time:	Cook Time:	Serving:	Beverage pairing:
15 min	0 min	1	Black Coffee

Ingredients:

- 1 cup rolled oats
- 1/4 cup almond butter (unsweetened)
- 1/4 cup dried cherries (unsweetened)
- 1/4 cup almonds, chopped
- 2 tablespoons honey (optional for sweetness)
- 1 tablespoon chia seeds

Preparation:

1. In a mixing bowl, combine all ingredients.
2. Mix until well combined and the mixture holds together.
3. Roll the mixture into small balls using your hands.
4. Place the energy bites on a tray lined with parchment paper.
5. Refrigerate for at least 30 minutes before serving.

Nutrient Facts (per serving):

- Calories: Approximately 100 per serving
- Carbohydrates: 8g
- Fat: 6g
- Protein: 4g

12. Sugar-Free Pickles

Prep.Time: 5 min

Cook Time: 0 min

Serving: 1

Beverage pairing: Mint Water

Ingredients:

- 1 cup sliced cucumbers
- 1/2 cup water
- 1/2 cup vinegar
- 1 tablespoon salt
- 1 teaspoon stevia (or other sugar substitute)
- 1/2 teaspoon dill (optional)

Preparation:

1. In a jar, combine water, vinegar, salt, stevia, and dill (if using). Stir until the salt and stevia are dissolved.
2. Add the sliced cucumbers to the jar.
3. Seal the jar and refrigerate for at least 24 hours before serving.

Nutrient Facts (per serving):

- Calories: Approximately 5 per serving
- Carbohydrates: 1g
- Fat: 0g
- Protein: 0g

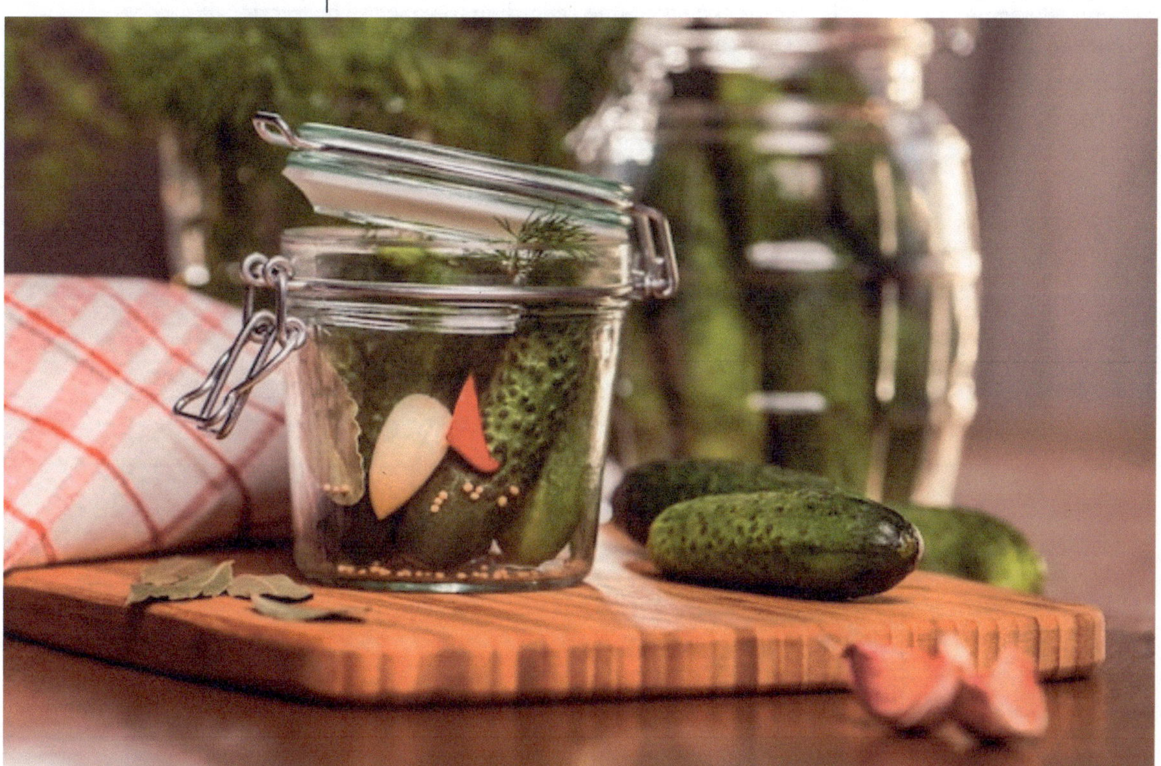

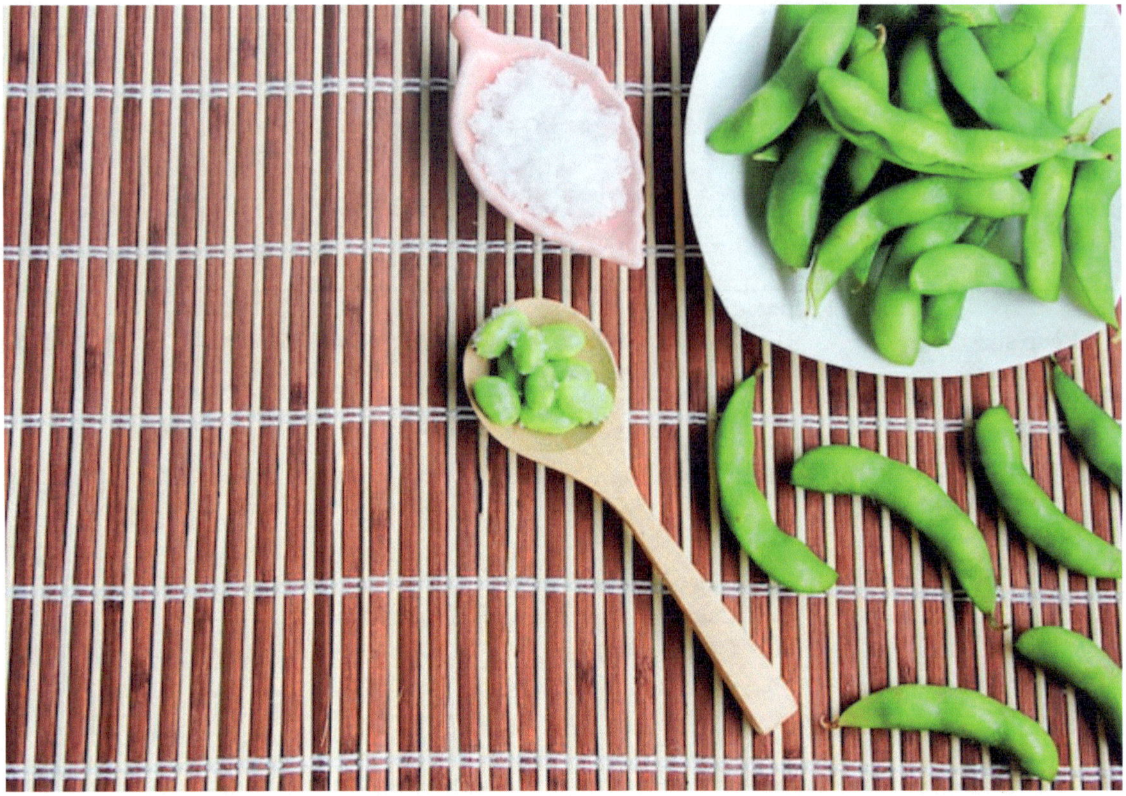

13. Edamame with a Dash of Sea Salt

Prep.Time:	Cook Time:	Serving:	Beverage pairing:
10 min	5 min	1	Cucumber Water

Ingredients:

- 1 cup edamame (cooked and shelled)
- Sea salt to taste

Preparation:

1. Cook the edamame according to package instructions.
2. Drain and rinse with cold water.
3. Sprinkle with sea salt to taste.

Nutrient Facts (per serving):

- Calories: Approximately 100 per serving
- Carbohydrates: 9g
- Fat: 4g
- Protein: 9g

14. Turkey and Cheese Roll-Ups

Prep.Time: 5 min

Cook Time: 0 min

Serving: 1

Beverage pairing: Black Coffee

Ingredients:

- 2 slices turkey breast
- 2 slices cheese (such as Swiss or cheddar)

Preparation:

1. Lay the turkey slices flat.
2. Place a slice of cheese on each turkey slice.
3. Roll up tightly and secure with a toothpick if needed.

Nutrient Facts (per serving):

- Calories: Approximately 150 per serving
- Carbohydrates: 2g
- Fat: 8g
- Protein: 16g

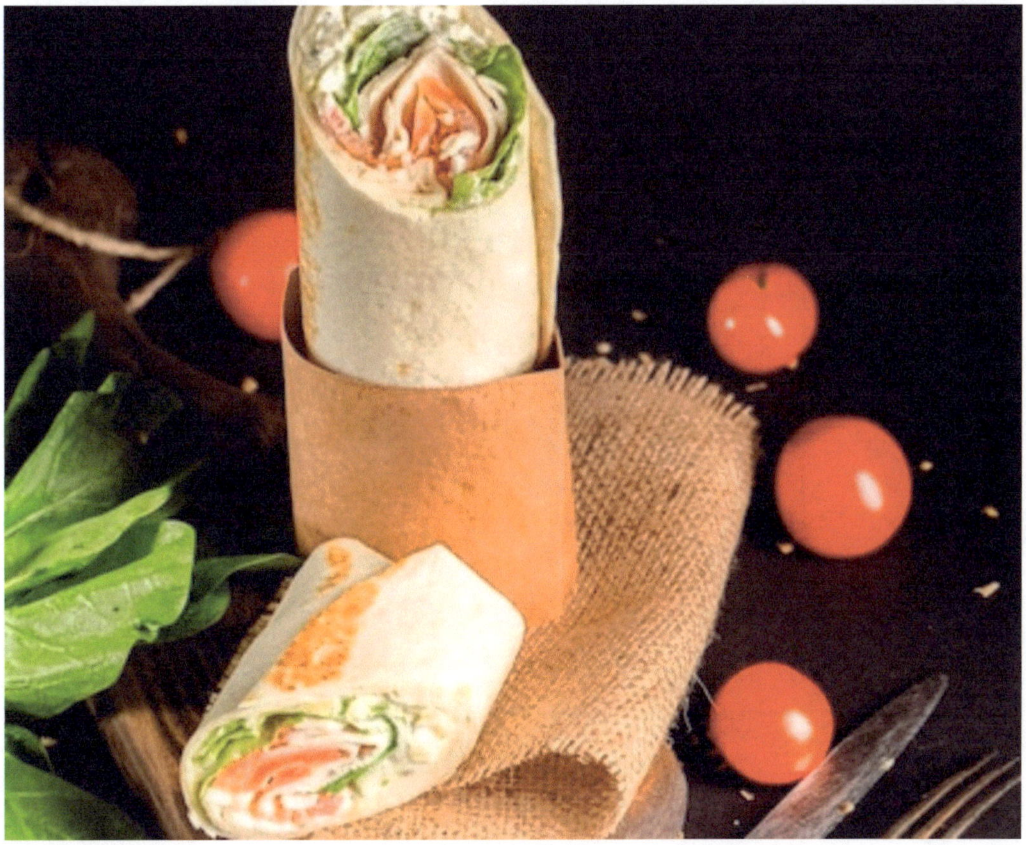

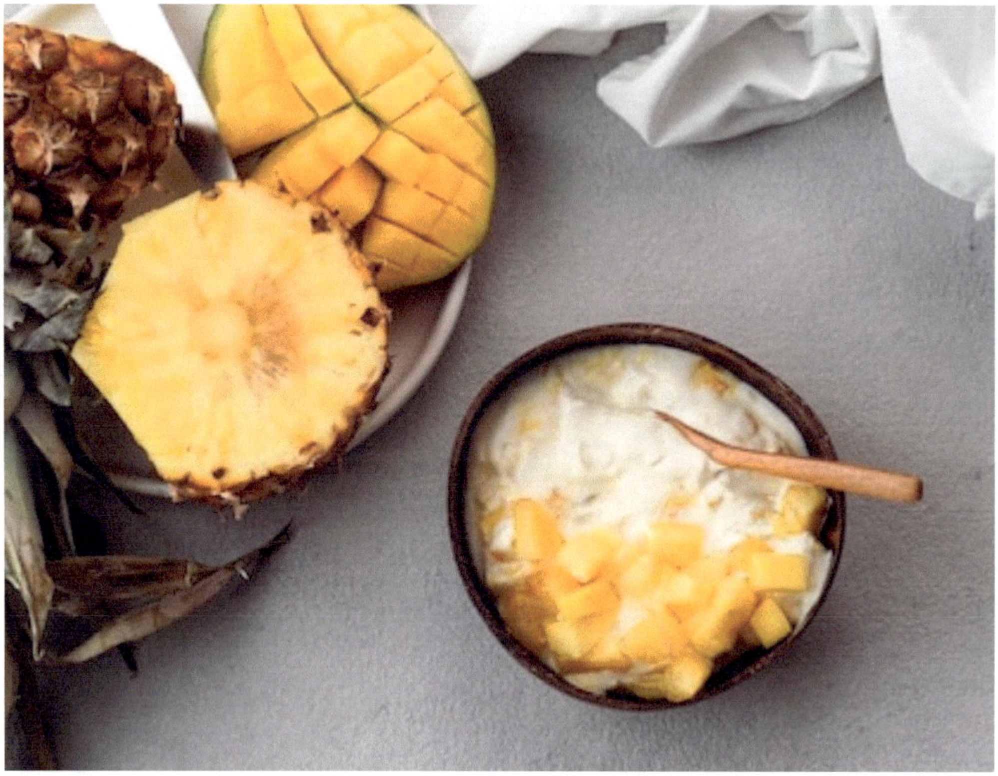

15. Cottage Cheese with Pineapple Chunks

Prep.Time: 5 min	Cook Time: 0 min	Serving: 1	Beverage pairing: Herbal Tea

Ingredients:

- 1/2 cup cottage cheese (low-fat or non-fat)
- 1/2 cup pineapple chunks (unsweetened)

Preparation:

1. In a bowl, combine cottage cheese and pineapple chunks.
2. Stir gently to mix.

Nutrient Facts (per serving):

- Calories: Approximately 150 per serving
- Carbohydrates: 14g
- Fat: 3g
- Protein: 15g

16. Roasted Chickpeas with Paprika

Prep.Time:	**Cook Time:**	**Serving:**	**Beverage pairing:**
5 min	25-30 min	1	Chamomile Tea

Ingredients:

- 1 can (15 ounces) chickpeas, drained and rinsed
- 1 tablespoon olive oil
- 1 teaspoon paprika
- Salt to taste

Preparation:

1. Preheat the oven to 400°F (200°C).
2. Pat the chickpeas dry with a paper towel.
3. In a bowl, toss chickpeas with olive oil, paprika, and salt until coated.
4. Spread the chickpeas on a baking sheet in a single layer.
5. Roast in the preheated oven for 25-30 minutes, or until crispy, shaking the pan occasionally.
6. Let cool before serving.

Nutrient Facts (per serving):

- Calories: Approximately 150 per serving
- Carbohydrates: 25g
- Fat: 3g
- Protein: 6g

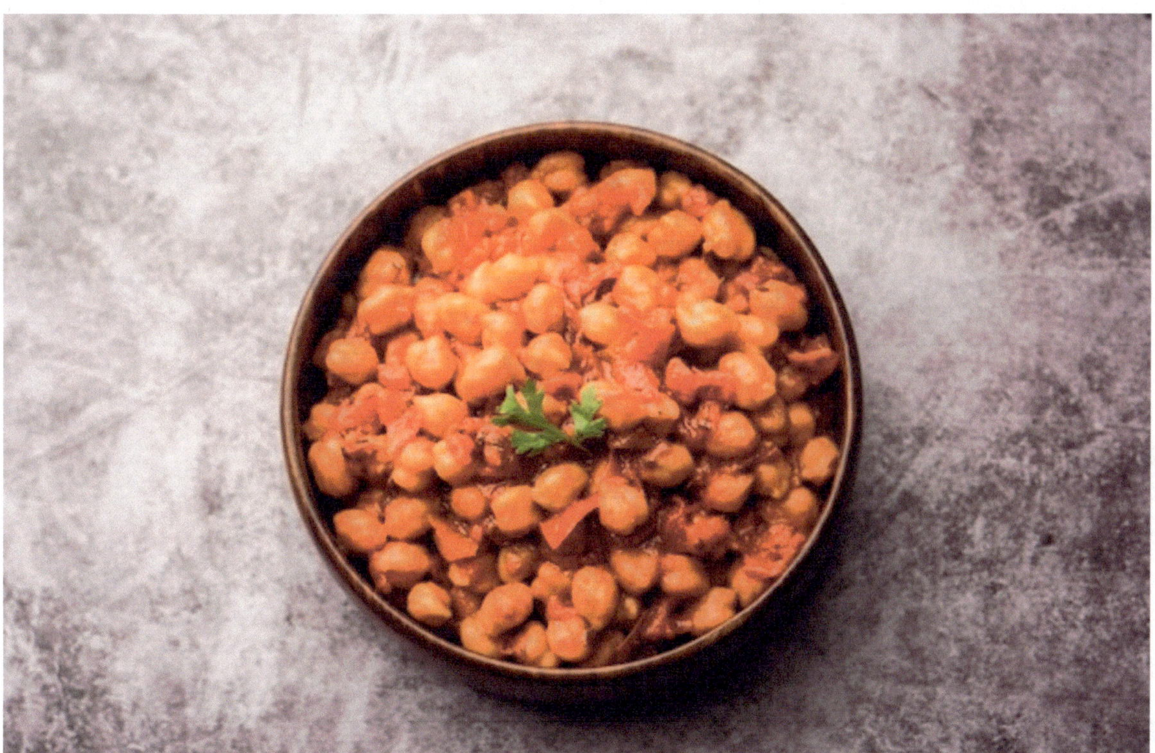

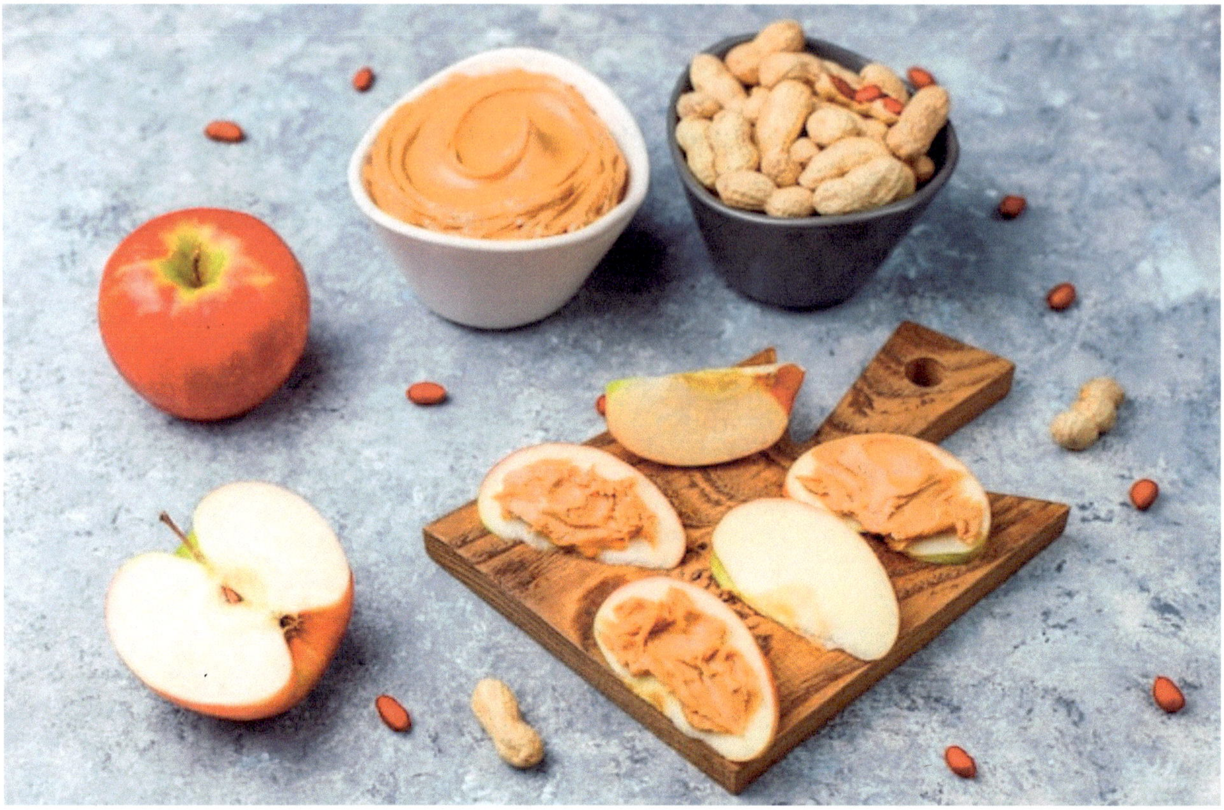

17. Apple Slices with Almond Butter

Prep.Time:	Cook Time:	Serving:	Beverage pairing:
5 min	0 min	1	Black Coffee

Ingredients:

- 1 medium apple, sliced
- 2 tablespoons almond butter (unsweetened)

Preparation:

1. Slice the apple into wedges.
2. Serve with almond butter for dipping.

Nutrient Facts (per serving):

- Calories: Approximately 150 per serving
- Carbohydrates: 20g
- Fat: 8g
- Protein: 3g

18. Seaweed Snacks

Prep.Time:	Cook Time:	Serving:	Beverage pairing:
0 min	0 min	1	Herbal Tea

Ingredients:

- Seaweed snack sheets

Preparation:

1. Simply open the package and enjoy!

Nutrient Facts (per serving):

- Calories: Approximately 30 per serving
- Carbohydrates: 1g
- Fat: 2g
- Protein: 1g

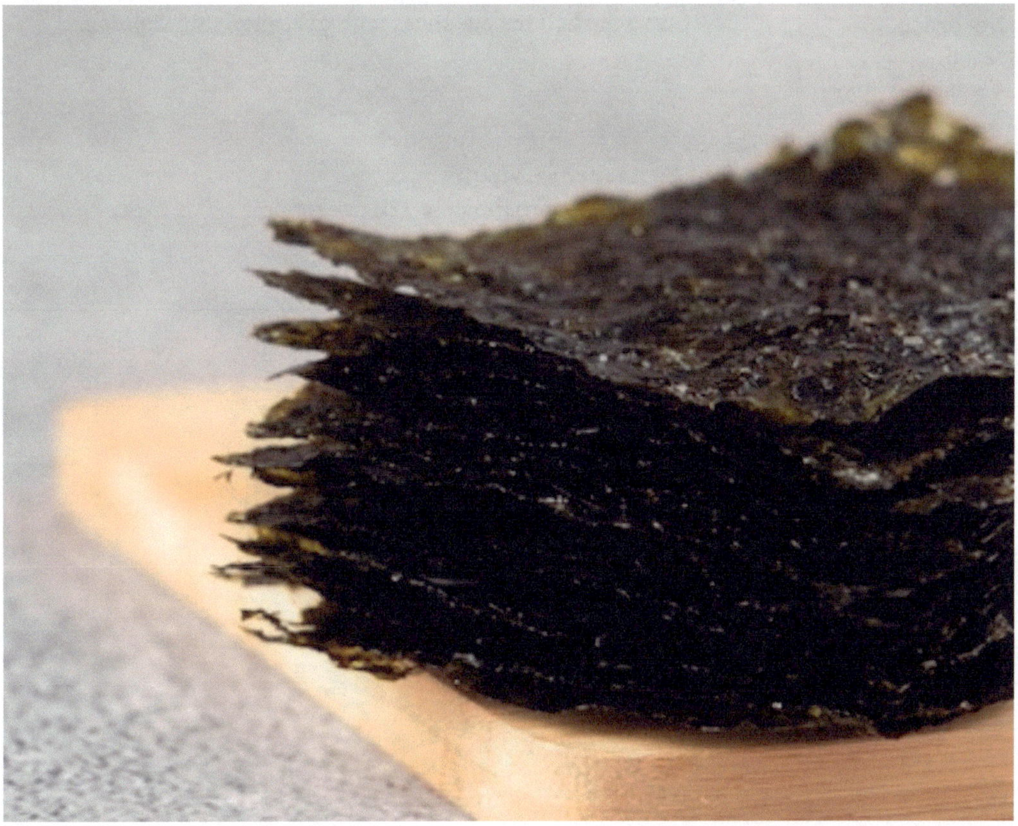

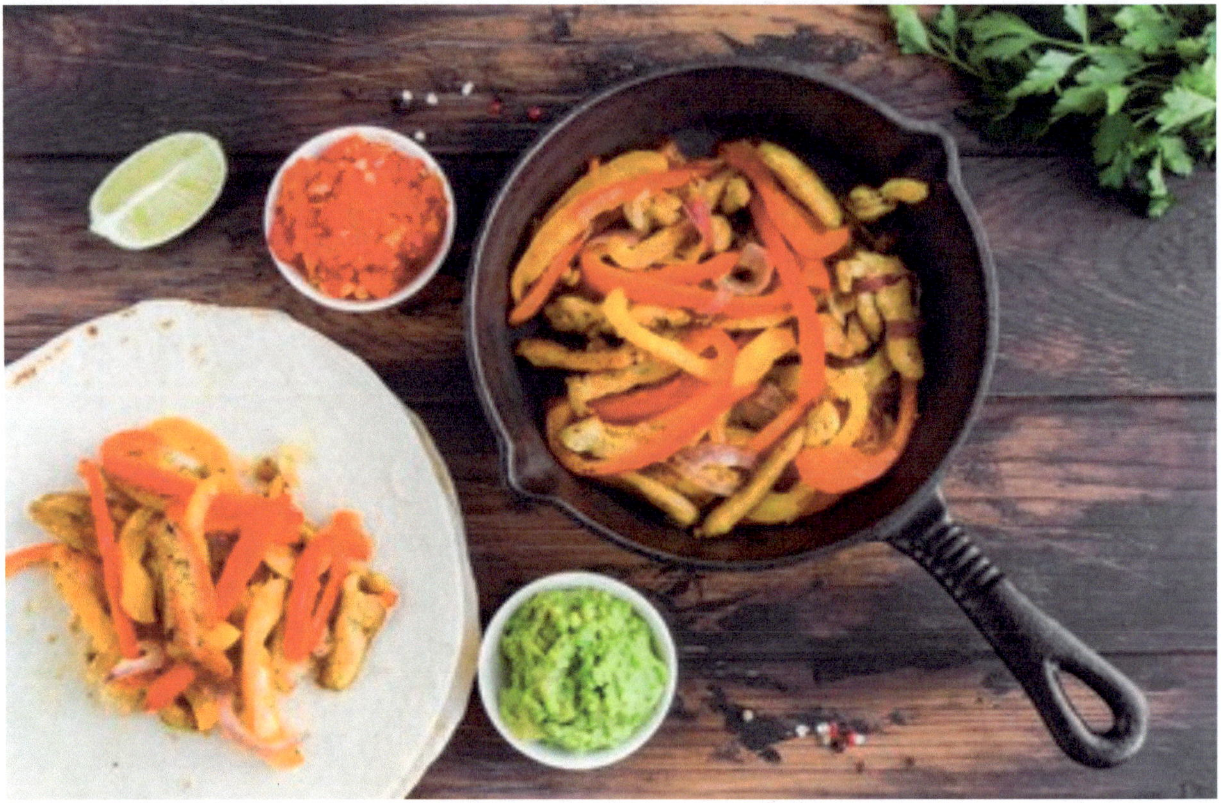

19. Sliced Bell Peppers with Guacamole

Prep.Time: 5 min

Cook Time: 0 min

Serving: 1

Beverage pairing: Green Tea

Ingredients:

- 1 bell pepper, sliced
- 1/2 avocado, mashed
- 1/4 teaspoon lime juice
- Salt and pepper to taste

Preparation:

1. Slice the bell pepper into strips.
2. In a bowl, mash the avocado and mix with lime juice, salt, and pepper.
3. Serve the bell pepper slices with guacamole for dipping.

Nutrient Facts (per serving):

- Calories: Approximately 120 per serving
- Carbohydrates: 8g
- Fat: 9g
- Protein: 2g

20. Yogurt-Covered Almonds

Prep.Time:	Cook Time:	Serving:	Beverage pairing:
10 min	0 min	1	Water

Ingredients:

- 1/4 cup almonds
- 1/4 cup Greek yogurt (unsweetened)

Preparation:

1. Dip each almond into Greek yogurt until coated.
2. Place on a parchment-lined tray.
3. Freeze for 1-2 hours until yogurt is set.

Nutrient Facts (per serving):

- Calories: Approximately 150 per serving
- Carbohydrates: 15g
- Fat: 8g
- Protein: 6g

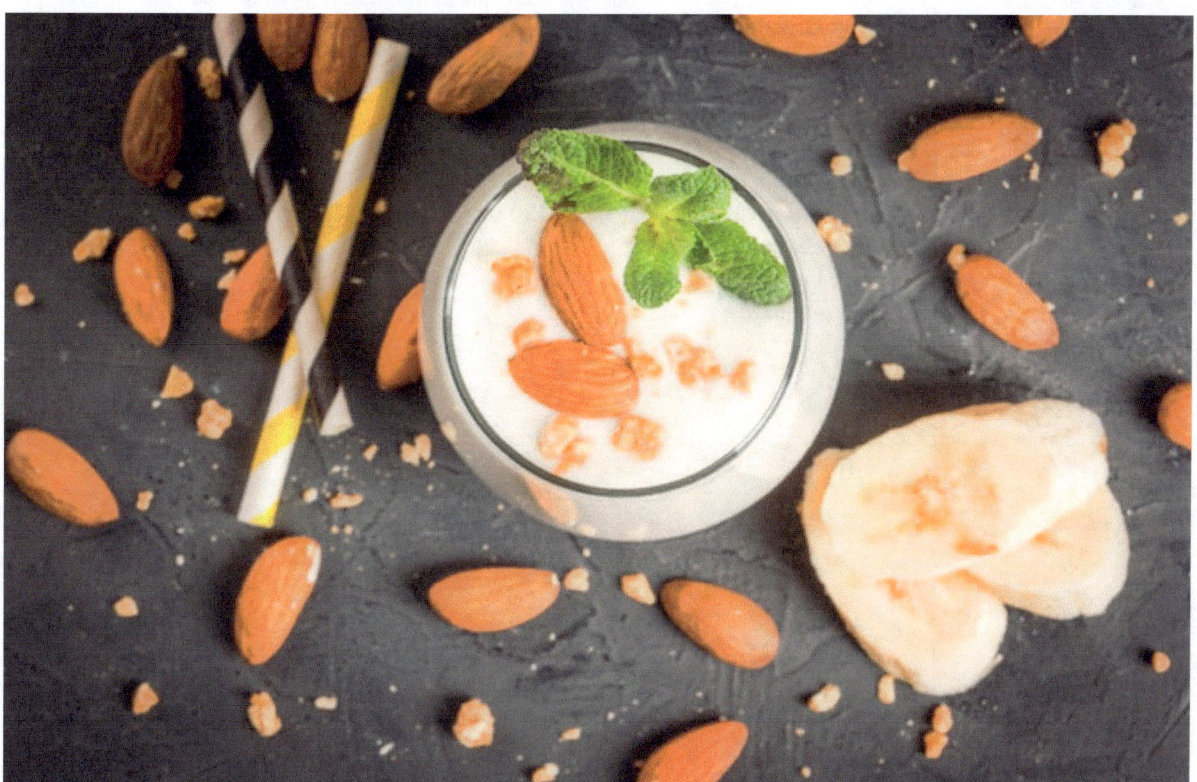

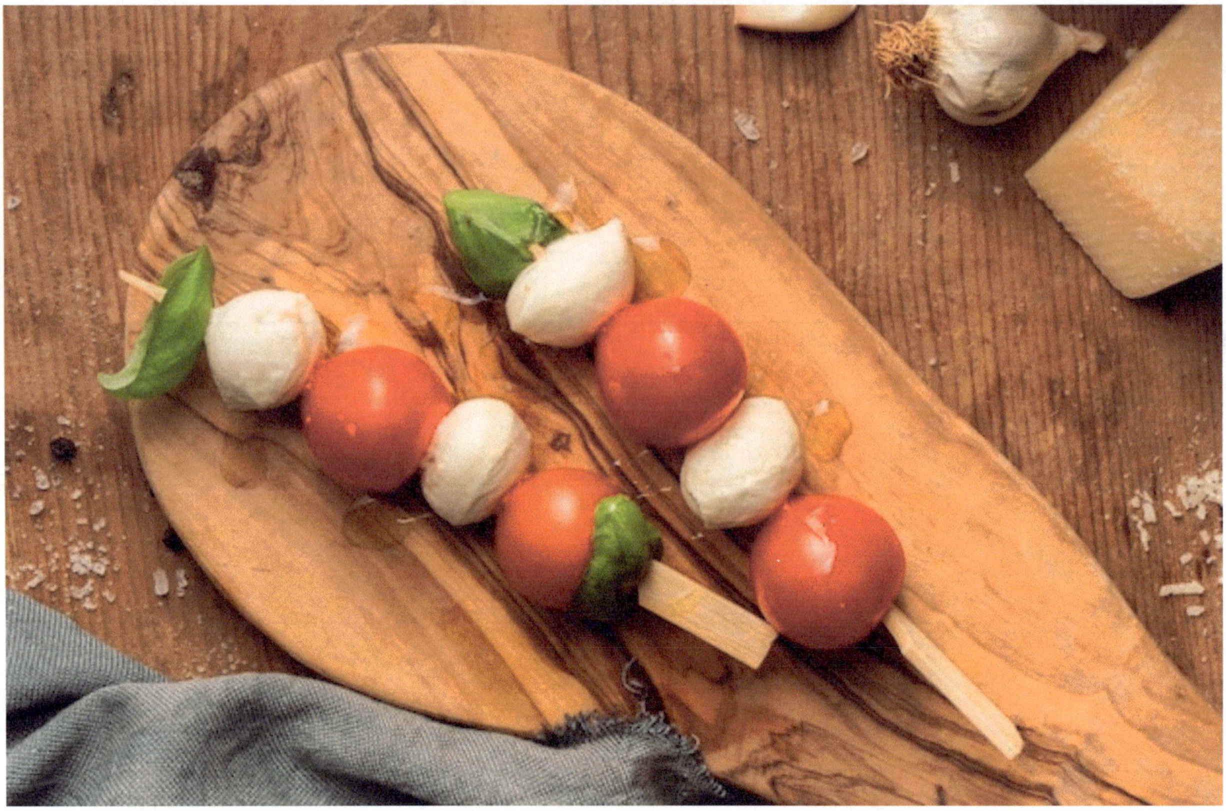

21. Tomato and Mozzarella Caprese Skewers

Prep.Time: 10 min

Cook Time: 0 min

Serving: 1

Beverage pairing: Black Coffee

Ingredients:

- Cherry tomatoes
- Fresh mozzarella balls
- Basil leaves
- Balsamic glaze (optional)

Preparation:

1. Thread cherry tomatoes, mozzarella balls, and basil leaves onto skewers.
2. Drizzle with balsamic glaze if desired.

Nutrient Facts (per serving):

- Calories: Approximately 120 per serving
- Carbohydrates: 3g
- Fat: 9g
- Protein: 7g

22. Cinnamon Roasted Pumpkin Seeds

Prep.Time:	Cook Time:	Serving:	Beverage pairing:
10 min	30 min	1	Herbal Tea

Ingredients:

- 1 cup pumpkin seeds
- 1 tablespoon olive oil
- 1 tablespoon maple syrup (sugar-free)
- 1 teaspoon ground cinnamon
- Pinch of salt

Preparation:

1. Preheat the oven to 300°F (150°C).
2. In a bowl, toss pumpkin seeds with olive oil, maple syrup, cinnamon, and salt until coated.
3. Spread the pumpkin seeds on a baking sheet in a single layer.
4. Roast in the preheated oven for 30-40 minutes, stirring occasionally, until golden and crispy.
5. Let cool before serving.

Nutrient Facts (per serving):

- Calories: Approximately 150 per serving
- Carbohydrates: 4g
- Fat: 12g
- Protein: 6g

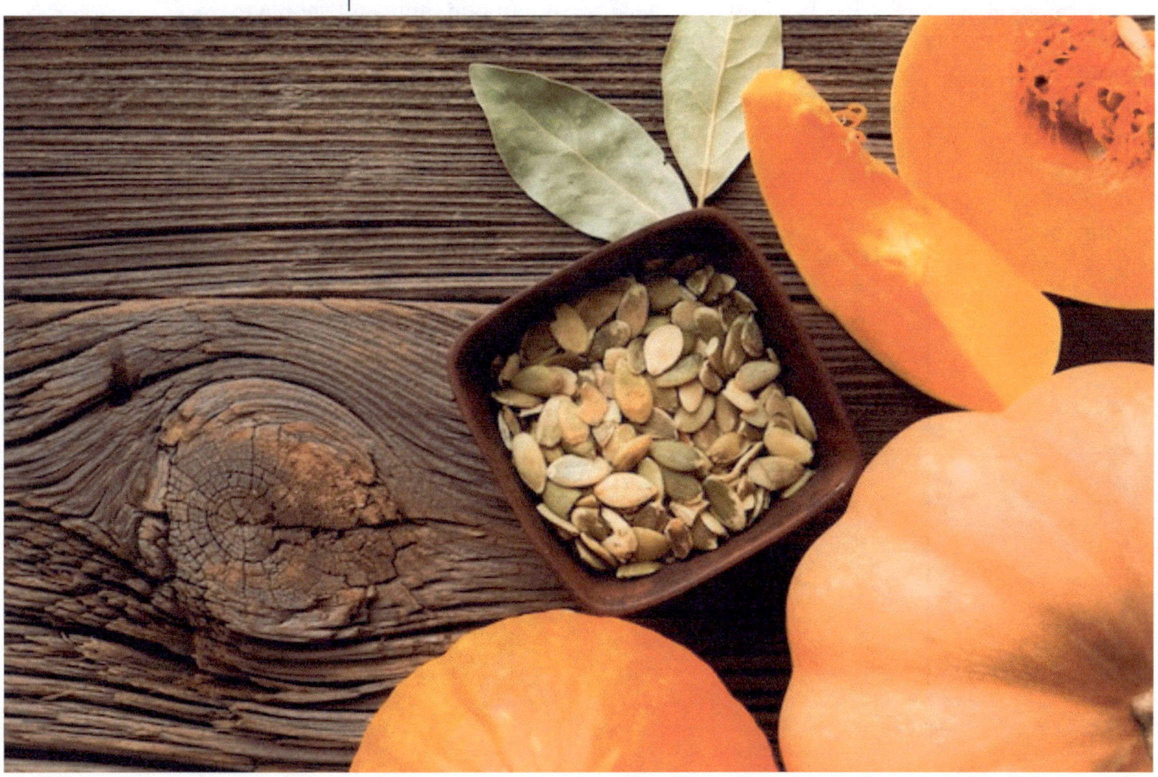

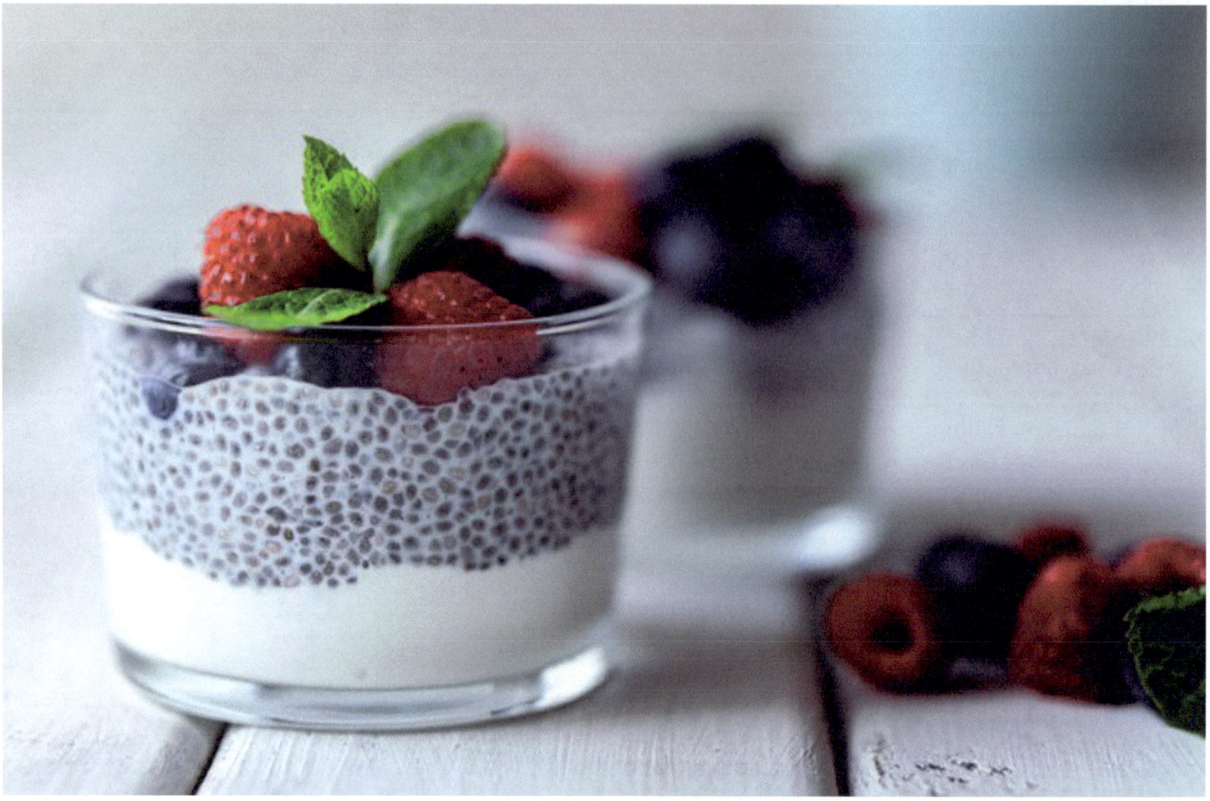

23. Chia Seed Pudding with Berries

Prep.Time: 5 min | **Cook Time:** 0 min | **Serving:** 1 | **Beverage pairing:** Black Coffee

Ingredients:

- 2 tablespoons chia seeds
- 1/2 cup unsweetened almond milk
- 1/4 teaspoon vanilla extract
- 1/2 cup mixed berries

Preparation:

1. In a bowl, mix chia seeds, almond milk, and vanilla extract.
2. Let the mixture sit for at least 30 minutes or overnight in the refrigerator until thickened.
3. Serve with mixed berries on top.

Nutrient Facts (per serving):

- Calories: Approximately 150 per serving
- Carbohydrates: 20g
- Fat: 7g
- Protein: 5g

24. Veggies and Salsa Dip

Prep.Time: 10 min	Cook Time: 0 min	Serving: 1	Beverage pairing: Orange Juice

Ingredients:

- Assorted sliced vegetables (carrots, celery, bell peppers, cucumber)
- Sugar-free salsa

Preparation:

1. Wash and slice the vegetables.
2. Serve with salsa for dipping.

Nutrient Facts (per serving):

- Calories: Approximately 50 per serving
- Carbohydrates: 10g
- Fat: 0g
- Protein: 2g

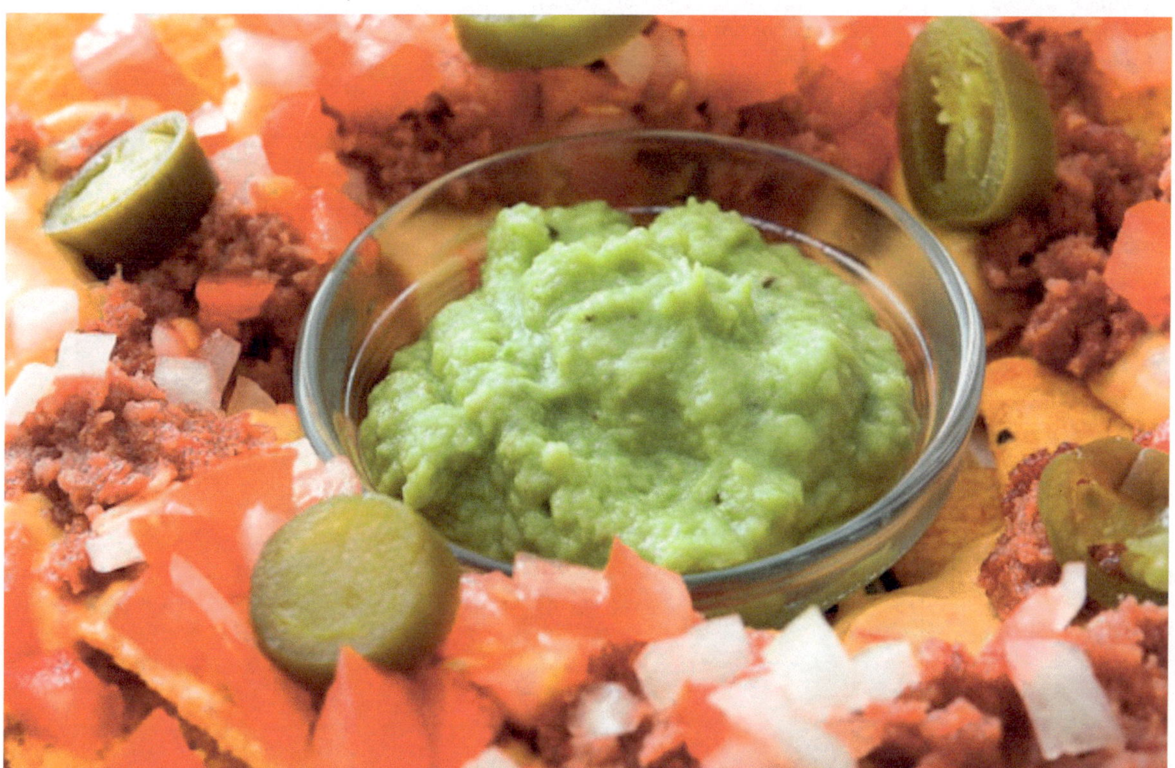

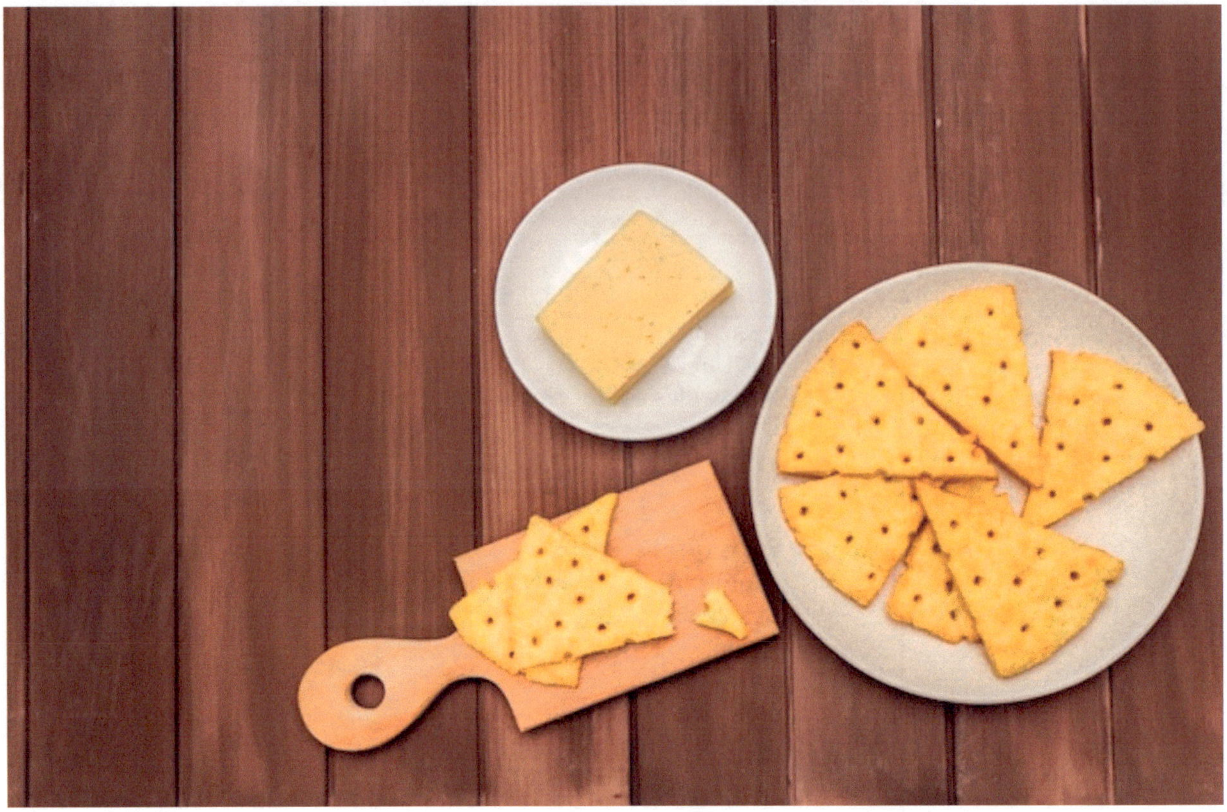

25. Cheese and Whole Grain Crackers

Prep.Time:	Cook Time:	Serving:	Beverage pairing:
5 min	0 min	1	Tea

Ingredients:

- 1 ounce cheese (such as cheddar or Swiss)
- 5-6 whole grain crackers

Preparation:

1. Cut the cheese into cubes.
2. Serve with whole grain crackers.

Nutrient Facts (per serving):

- Calories: Approximately 150 per serving
- Carbohydrates: 10g
- Fat: 9g
- Protein: 7g

26. Sliced Radishes with Cream Cheese

Prep.Time:	Cook Time:	Serving:	Beverage pairing:
5 min	0 min	1	Grapefruit Juice

Ingredients:

- 4-5 radishes, sliced
- 2 tablespoons cream cheese (low-fat or non-fat)

Preparation:

1. Wash and slice the radishes.
2. Spread cream cheese on each radish slice.

Nutrient Facts (per serving):

- Calories: Approximately 70 per serving
- Carbohydrates: 2g
- Fat: 6g
- Protein: 2g

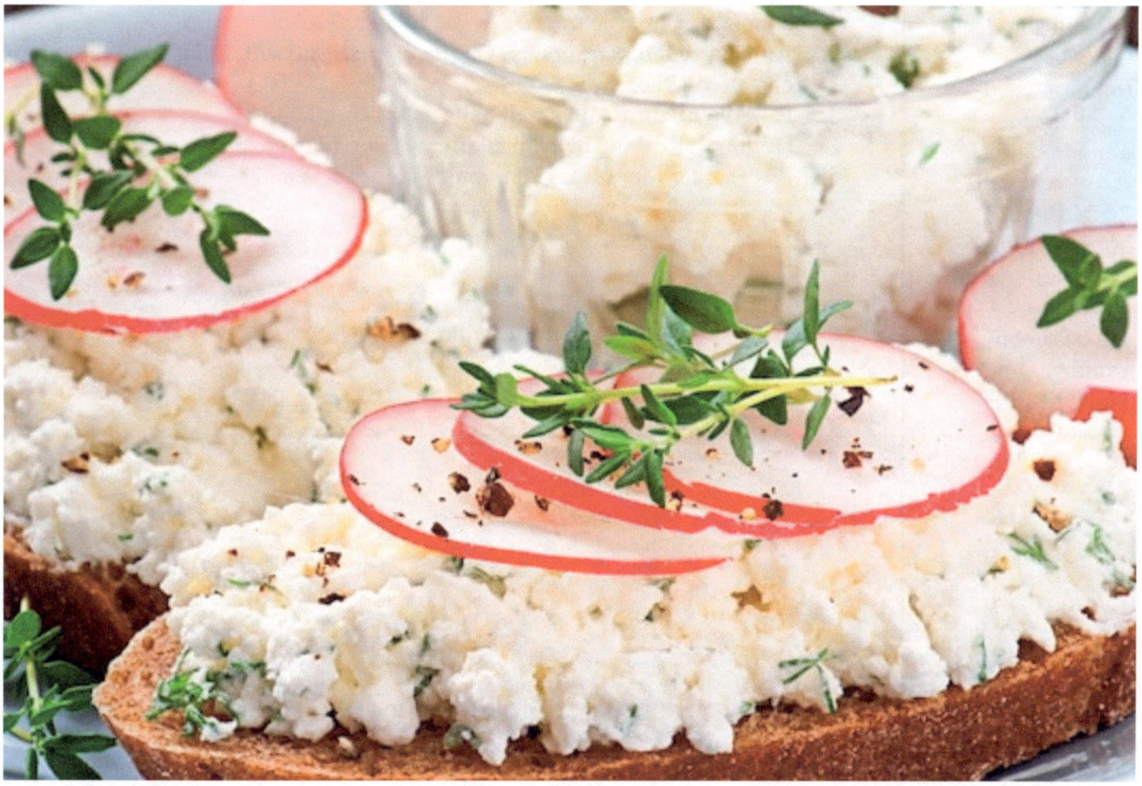

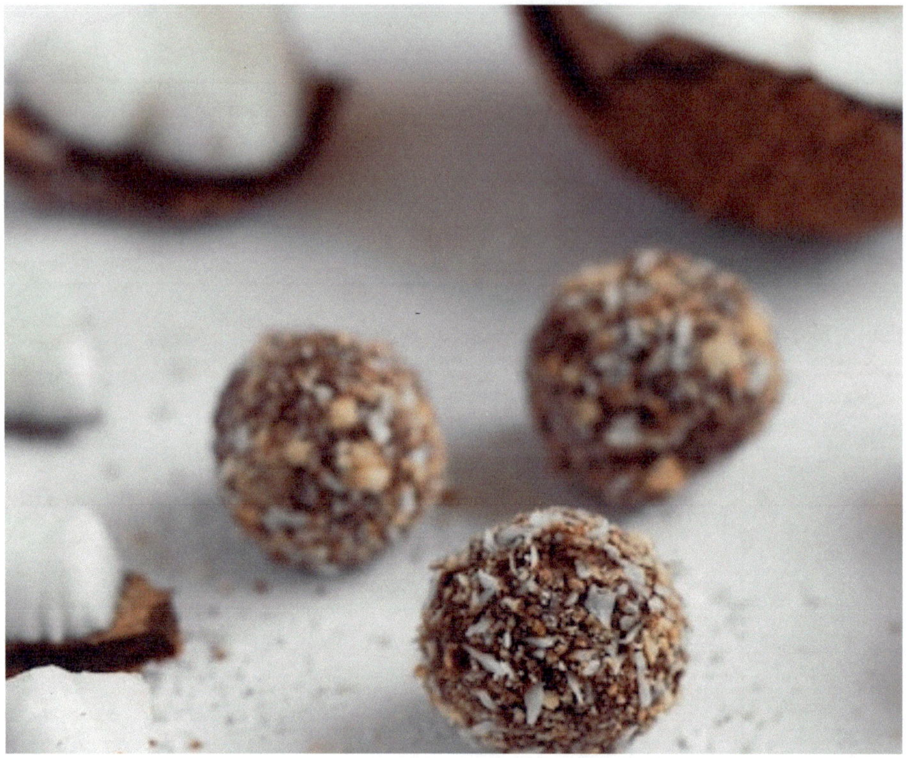

27. Almond and Coconut Energy Balls

Prep.Time:	Cook Time:	Serving:	Beverage pairing:
5 min	0 min	1	Black Cofee

Ingredients:

- 1/2 cup almonds
- 1/2 cup shredded coconut (unsweetened)
- 2 tablespoons almond butter (unsweetened)
- 2 tablespoons honey (or maple syrup for a vegan option)
- 1/2 teaspoon vanilla extract
- Pinch of salt

Preparation:

1. In a food processor, pulse almonds and shredded coconut until finely chopped.
2. Add almond butter, honey, vanilla extract, and salt. Pulse until the mixture comes together.
3. Roll the mixture into small balls using your hands.
4. Optional: Roll the balls in additional shredded coconut for coating.
5. Refrigerate for at least 30 minutes before serving.

Nutrient Facts (per serving):

- Calories: Approximately 120 per serving
- Carbohydrates: 10g
- Fat: 8g
- Protein: 4g

28. Spicy Roasted Nuts Mix

Prep.Time:	Cook Time:	Serving:	Beverage pairing:
5 min	10-15 min	1	Coffee

Ingredients:

- 1 cup mixed nuts (almonds, cashews, walnuts)
- 1 tablespoon olive oil
- 1 teaspoon chili powder
- 1/2 teaspoon paprika
- 1/4 teaspoon garlic powder
- Salt to taste

Preparation:

1. Preheat the oven to 350°F (175°C).
2. In a bowl, toss the mixed nuts with olive oil, chili powder, paprika, garlic powder, and salt until well coated.
3. Spread the nuts on a baking sheet in a single layer.
4. Roast in the preheated oven for 10-15 minutes, stirring halfway through, until golden and fragrant.
5. Let cool before serving.

Nutrient Facts (per serving):

- Calories: Approximately 160 per serving
- Carbohydrates: 5g
- Fat: 14g
- Protein: 6g

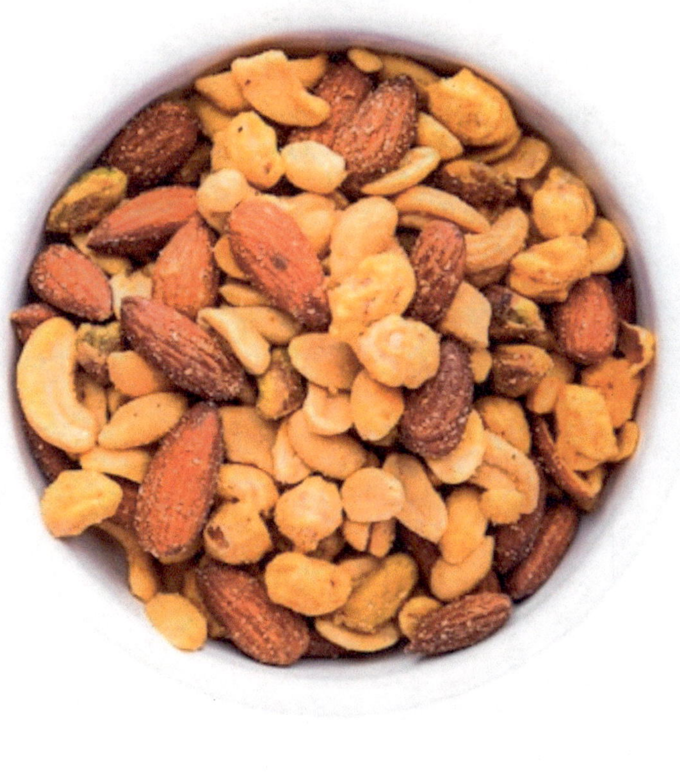

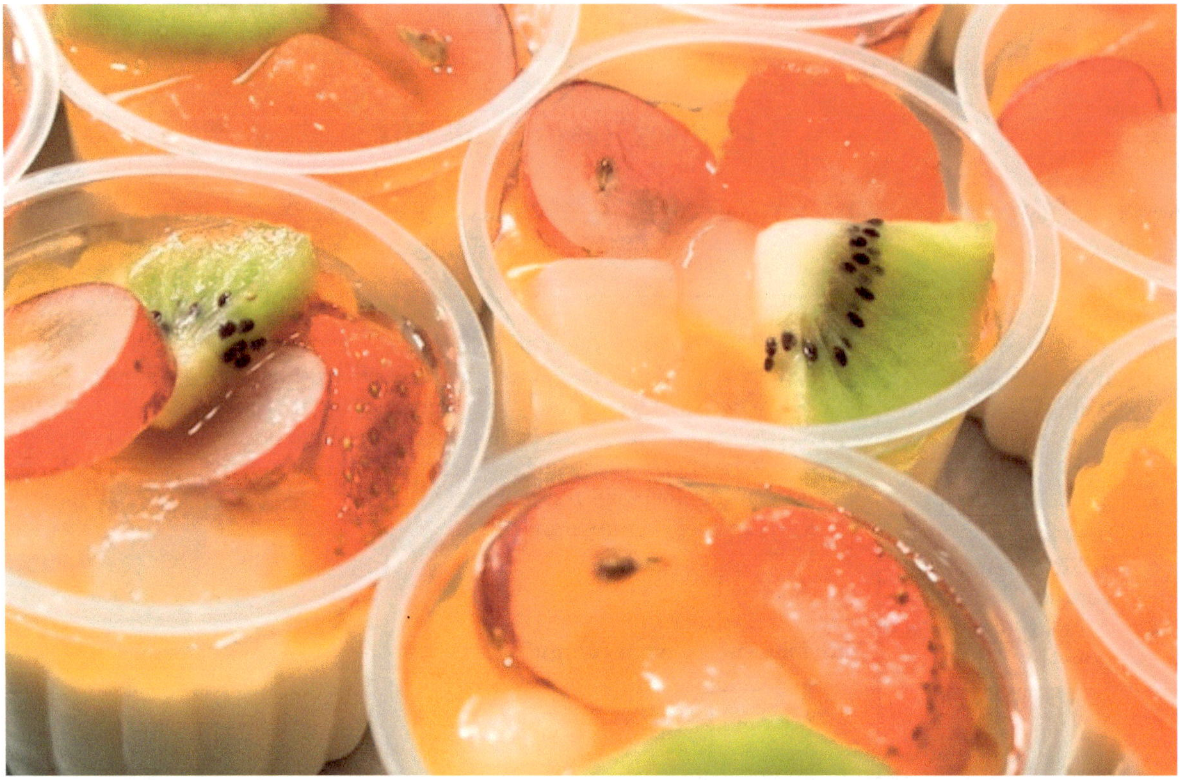

29. Sugar-Free Gelatin Cups with Fresh Fruit

Prep.Time: 5 min

Cook Time: 2-4 Hour

Serving: 1

Beverage pairing: Mint Water

Ingredients:

- Sugar-free gelatin cups (prepared according to package instructions)
- Assorted fresh fruits (such as berries, kiwi, pineapple)

Preparation:

1. Prepare the sugar-free gelatin according to package instructions and pour into cups.
2. Chill in the refrigerator until set.
3. Top with assorted fresh fruits before serving.

Nutrient Facts (per serving):

- Calories: Approximately 30 per serving
- Carbohydrates: 0g
- Fat: 0g
- Protein: 1g

30. Popcorn Seasoned with Herbs and Spices

Prep.Time: 10 min

Cook Time: 5 min

Serving: 1

Beverage pairing: Black Coffee

Ingredients:

- 1/4 cup popcorn kernels
- 1 tablespoon olive oil
- 1 teaspoon dried herbs (such as oregano, thyme, or rosemary)
- 1/2 teaspoon garlic powder
- Salt to taste

Preparation:

1. Heat the olive oil in a large pot over medium heat.
2. Add the popcorn kernels and cover with a lid.
3. Cook, shaking the pot occasionally, until the popping slows down.
4. Remove from heat and transfer to a large bowl.
5. In a small bowl, mix dried herbs, garlic powder, and salt.
6. Sprinkle the herb mixture over the popcorn and toss to coat evenly.

Nutrient Facts (per serving):

- Calories: Approximately 100 per serving
- Carbohydrates: 20g
- Fat: 2g
- Protein: 3g

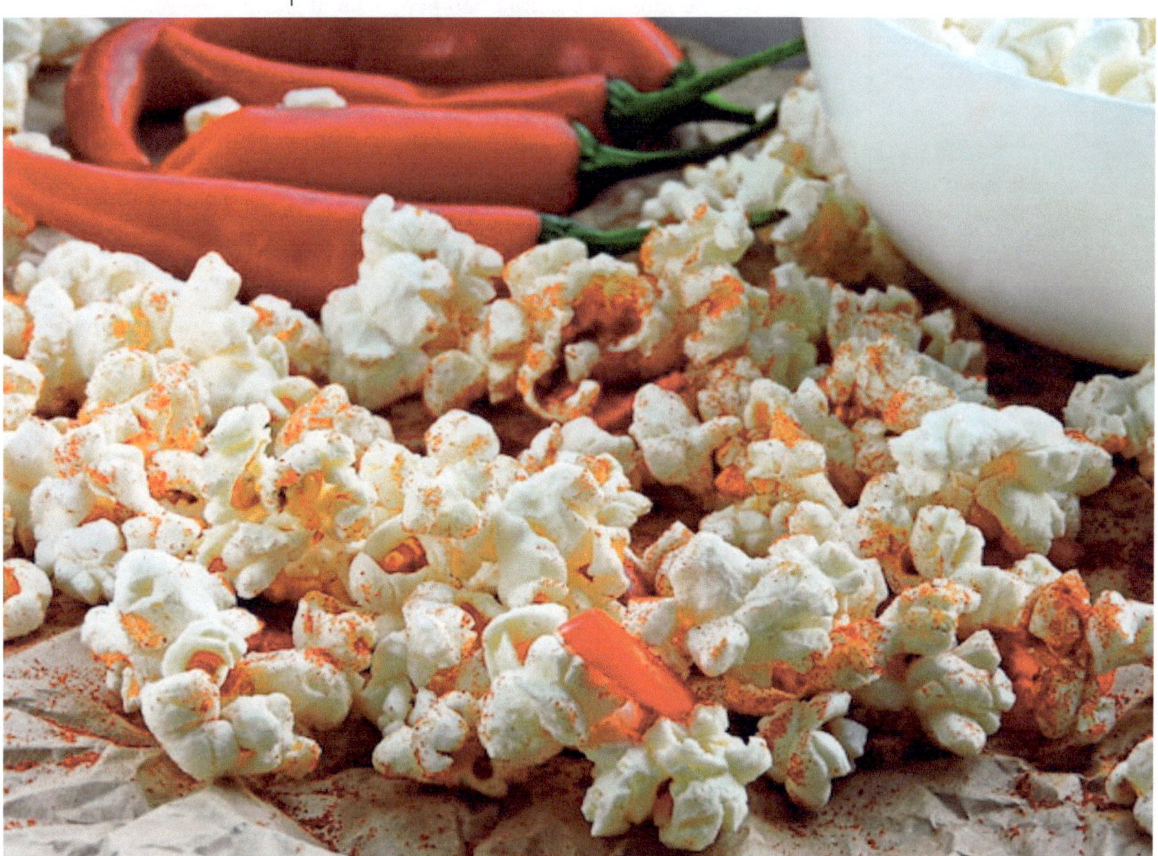

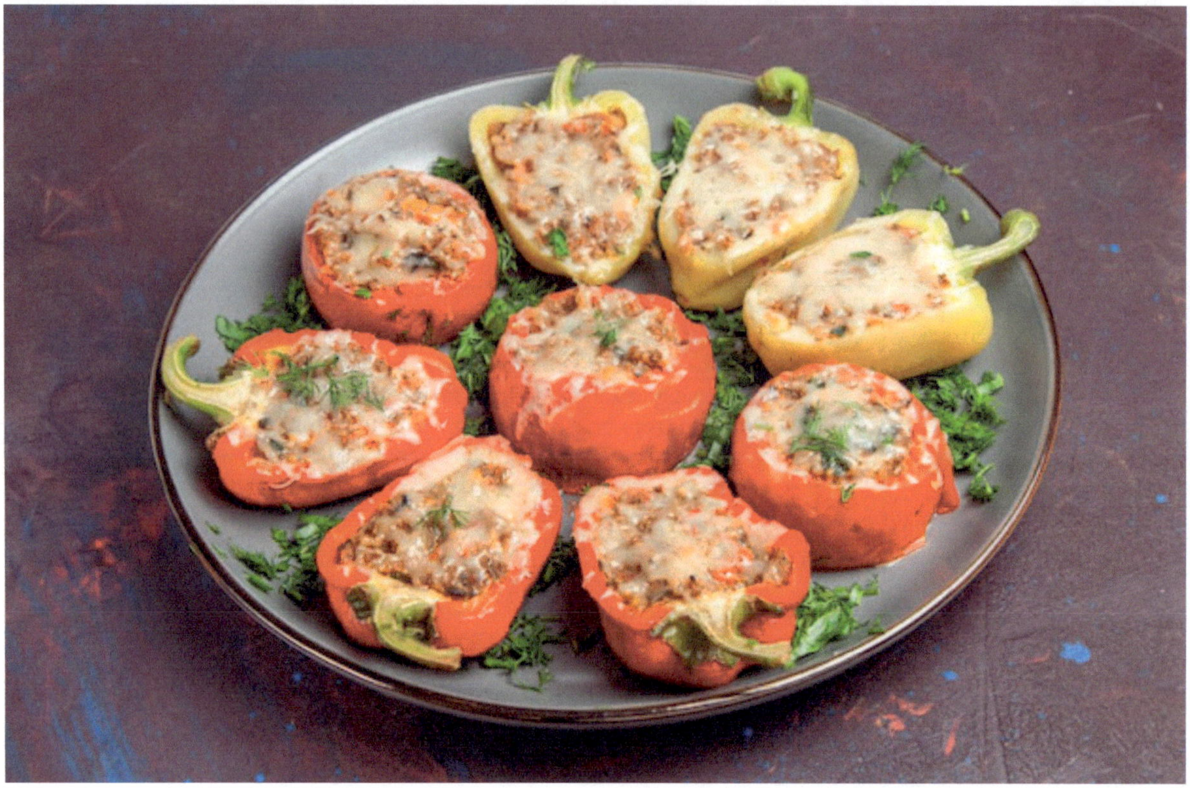

31. Stuffed Mini Bell Peppers with Cream Cheese

Prep.Time:	Cook Time:	Serving:	Beverage pairing:
10 min	0 min	1	Green Tea

Ingredients:

- Mini bell peppers
- Cream cheese (low-fat or non-fat)

Preparation:

1. Cut the tops off the mini bell peppers and remove the seeds.
2. Fill each pepper with cream cheese.
3. Serve immediately or refrigerate until ready to serve.

Nutrient Facts (per serving):

- Calories: Approximately 100 per serving
- Carbohydrates: 5g
- Fat: 8g
- Protein: 3g

32. Sliced Jicama with Lime and Chili Powder

Prep.Time: 10 min	**Cook Time:** 0 min	**Serving:** 1	**Beverage pairing:** Orange Juice

Ingredients:

- 1 small jicama, peeled and sliced
- Lime wedges
- Chili powder

Preparation:

1. Arrange jicama slices on a plate.
2. Squeeze lime juice over the slices.
3. Sprinkle with chili powder to taste.

Nutrient Facts (per serving):

- Calories: Approximately 50 per serving
- Carbohydrates: 12g
- Fat: 0g
- Protein: 1g

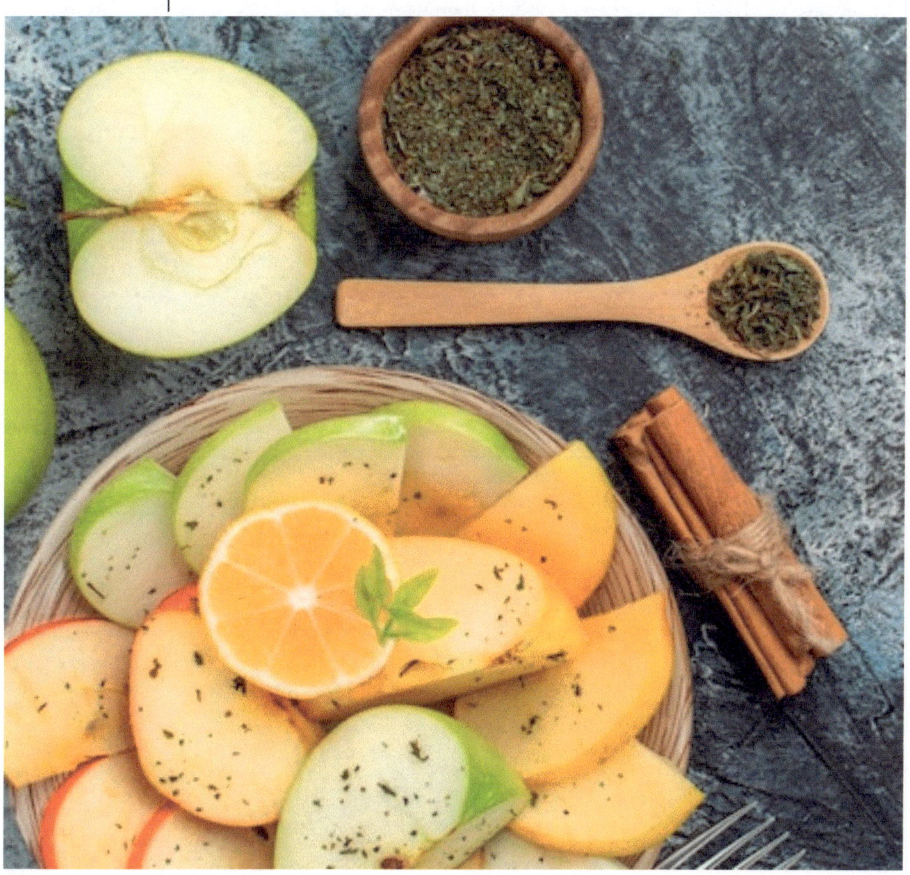

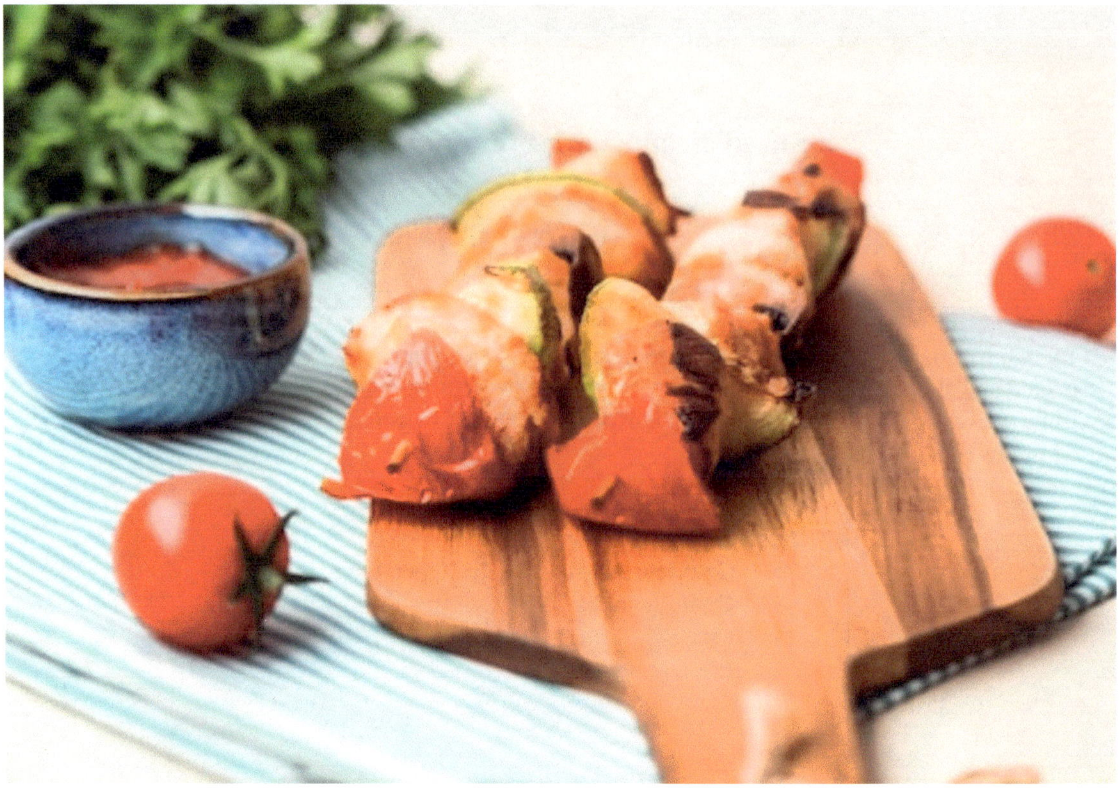

33. Cherry Tomato and Basil Skewers

Prep.Time:	Cook Time:	Serving:	Beverage pairing:
10 min	0 min	1	Black Coffee

Ingredients:

- Cherry tomatoes
- Fresh basil leaves
- Balsamic glaze (optional)

Preparation:

1. Thread cherry tomatoes and basil leaves onto skewers.
2. Drizzle with balsamic glaze if desired.

Nutrient Facts (per serving):

- Calories: Approximately 30 per serving
- Carbohydrates: 5g
- Fat: 0g
- Protein: 2g

34. Smoked Salmon Cucumber Bites

Prep.Time: 10 min	**Cook Time:** 0 min	**Serving:** 1	**Beverage pairing:** Mint Tea

Ingredients:

- Cucumber slices
- Smoked salmon slices
- Cream cheese (low-fat or non-fat)

Preparation:

1. Slice cucumber into rounds.
2. Spread cream cheese on each cucumber slice.
3. Top with a piece of smoked salmon.

Nutrient Facts (per serving):

- Calories: Approximately 70 per serving
- Carbohydrates: 2g
- Fat: 5g
  Protein: 5g

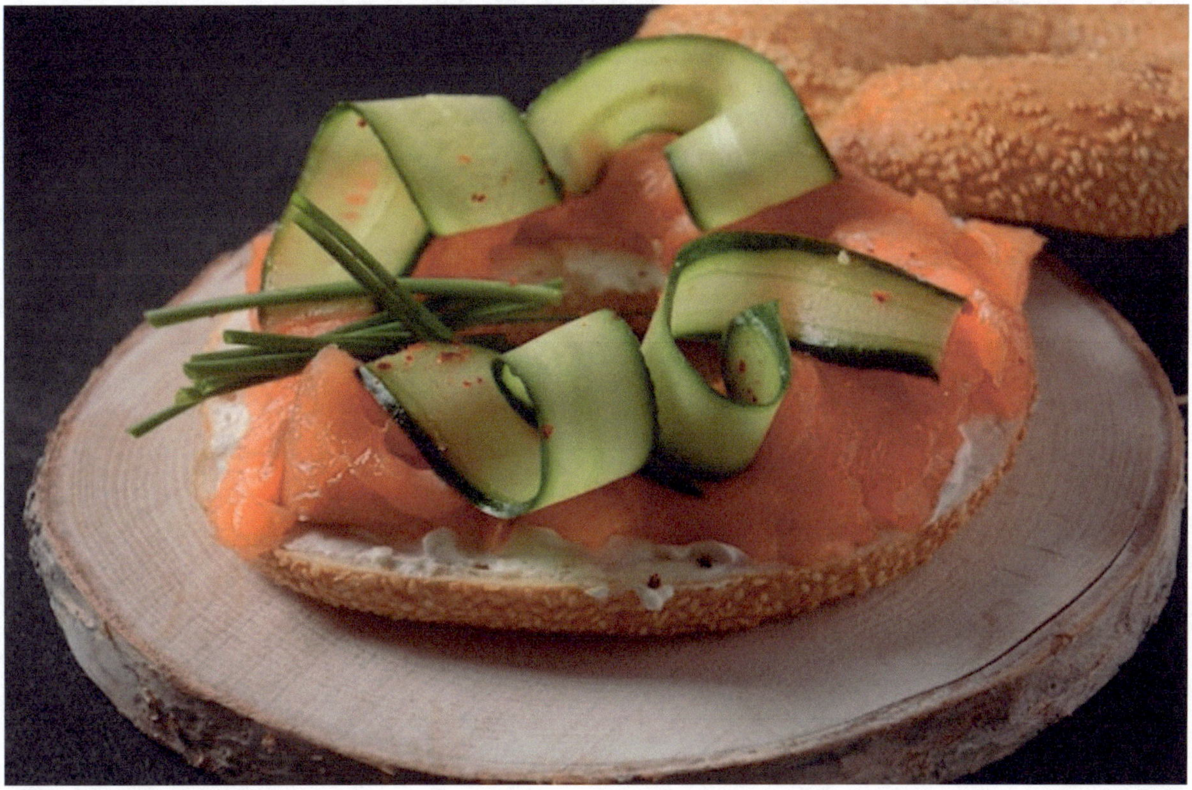

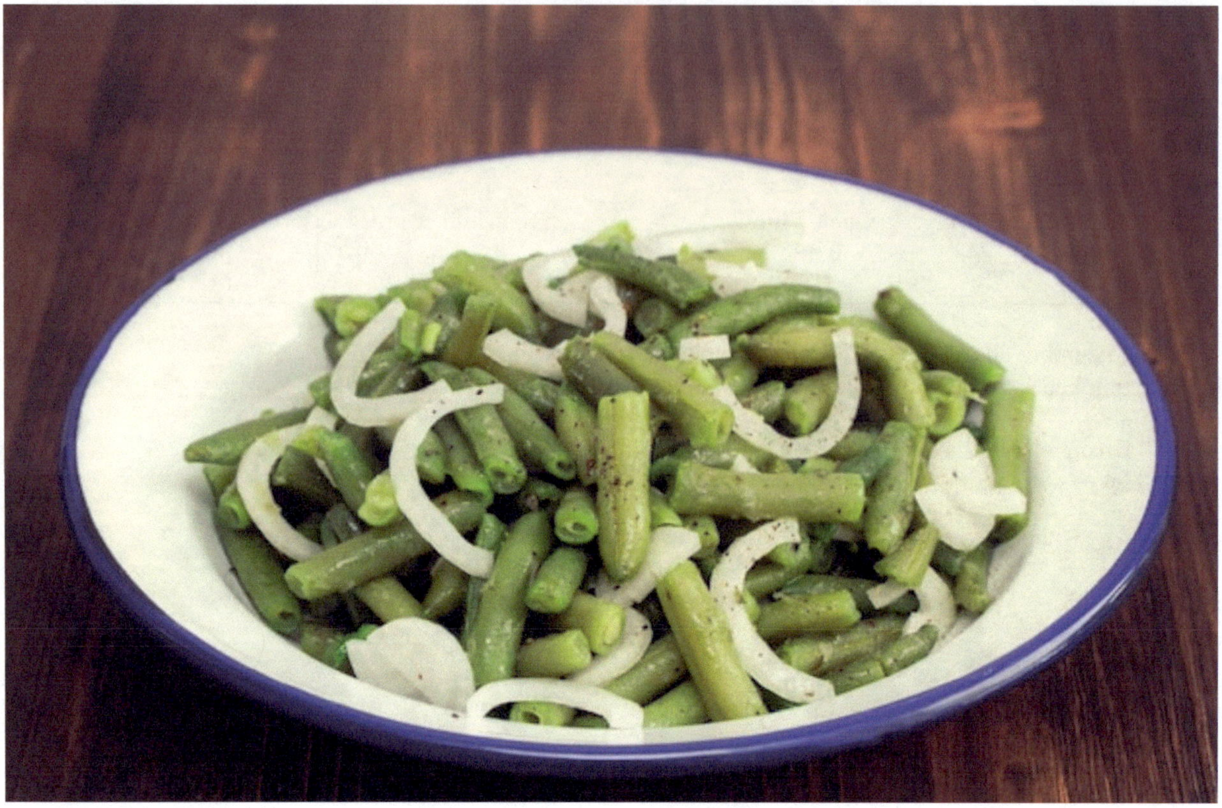

35. Green Bean Fries with Garlic Aioli

Prep.Time: 10 min

Cook Time: 15-20 min

Serving: 1

Beverage pairing: Lemonade

Ingredients:

- 1 pound fresh green beans, trimmed
- 2 tablespoons olive oil
- Salt and pepper to taste
- 1/4 cup mayonnaise (preferably sugar-free)
- 1 clove garlic, minced
- 1 teaspoon lemon juice

Preparation:

1. Preheat the oven to 425°F (220°C).
2. In a bowl, toss green beans with olive oil, salt, and pepper until coated.
3. Spread the green beans on a baking sheet in a single layer.
4. Roast in the preheated oven for 15-20 minutes, or until golden and crispy.
5. In a small bowl, mix mayonnaise, minced garlic, and lemon juice to make the garlic aioli.
6. Serve the green bean fries with the garlic aioli for dipping.

Nutrient Facts (per serving):

- Calories: Approximately 120 per serving
- Carbohydrates: 10g
- Fat: 8g
- Protein: 3g

36. Sugar-Free Yogurt with Chopped Nuts

Prep.Time: 2 min	**Cook Time:** 0 min	**Serving:** 1	**Beverage pairing:** Black Coffee

Ingredients:

- 1/2 cup sugar-free yogurt (such as Greek yogurt)
- 2 tablespoons chopped nuts (such as almonds, walnuts, or pecans)

Preparation:

1. Spoon the sugar-free yogurt into a bowl.
2. Sprinkle chopped nuts on top.

Nutrient Facts (per serving):

- Calories: Approximately 150 per serving
- Carbohydrates: 8g
- Fat: 10g
- Protein: 8g

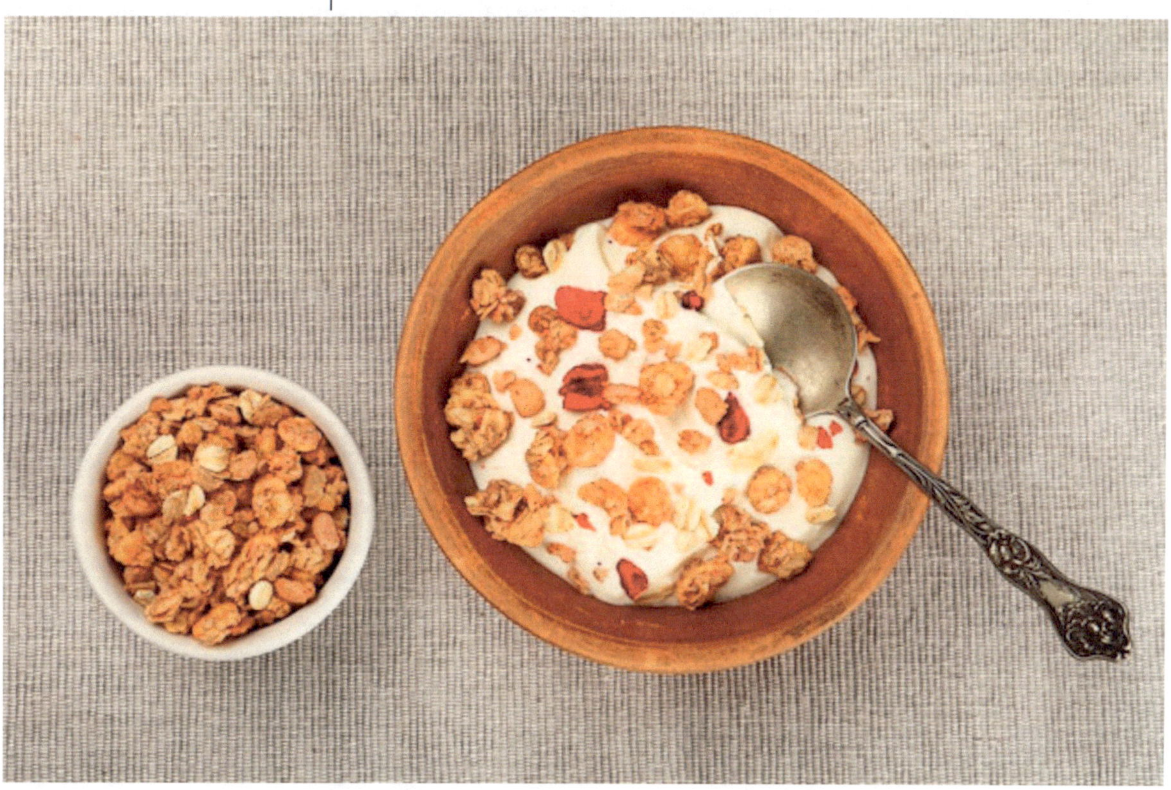

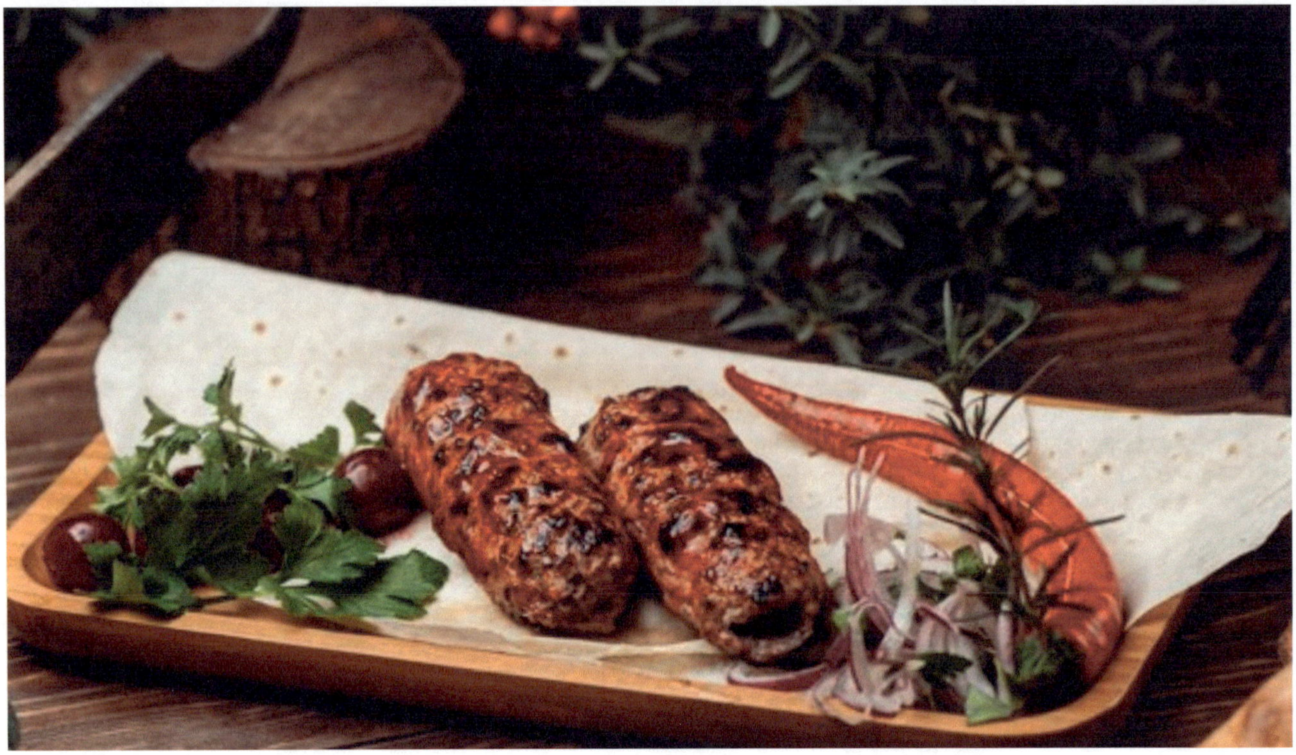

37. Mozzarella and Turkey Pepperoni Kabobs

Prep.Time: 5 min	**Cook Time:** 0 min	**Serving:** 1	**Beverage pairing:** Mint Tea

Ingredients:

- Mozzarella cheese balls
- Turkey pepperoni slices

Preparation:

1. Thread mozzarella cheese balls and turkey pepperoni slices onto skewers.

Nutrient Facts (per serving):

- Calories: Approximately 150 per serving
- Carbohydrates: 2g
- Fat: 10g
- Protein: 12g

38. Almond Flour Crackers with Cheese

Prep.Time:	Cook Time:	Serving:	Beverage pairing:
2 min	0 min	1	Black Coffee

Ingredients:

- Almond flour crackers
- Cheese slices (such as cheddar or Swiss)

Preparation:

1. Arrange almond flour crackers on a plate.
2. Top each cracker with a slice of cheese.

Nutrient Facts (per serving):

- Calories: Approximately 120 per serving
- Carbohydrates: 4g
- Fat: 9g
- Protein: 6g

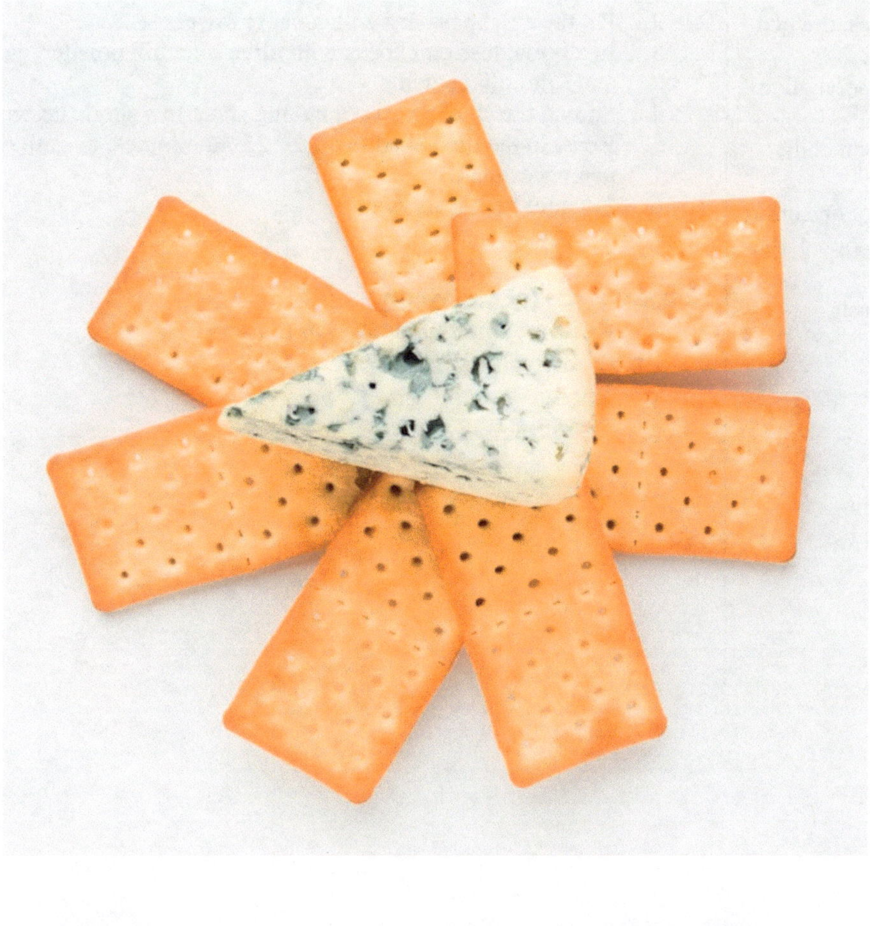

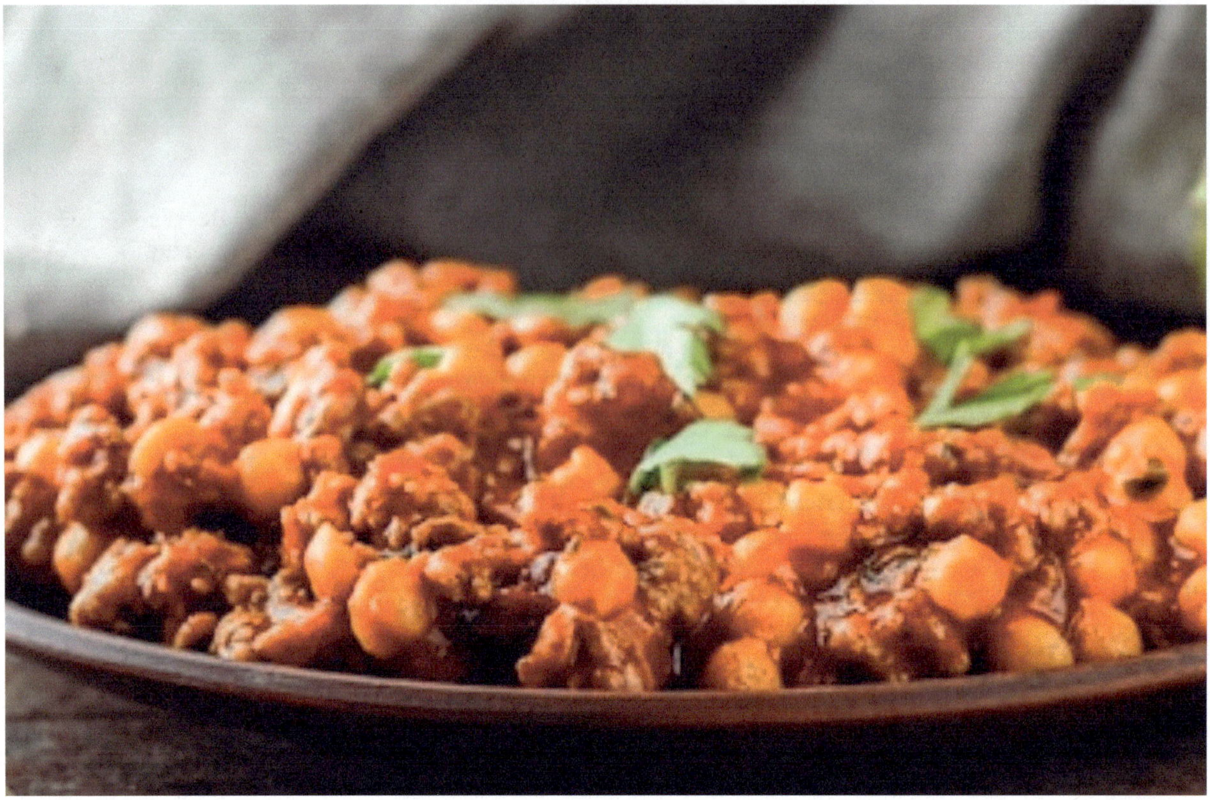

39. Spicy Roasted Chickpeas

Prep.Time:	Cook Time:	Serving:	Beverage pairing:
5 min	25-30 min	1	Tea

Ingredients:

- 1 can (15 ounces) chickpeas, drained and rinsed
- 1 tablespoon olive oil
- 1 teaspoon chili powder
- 1/2 teaspoon cumin
- 1/4 teaspoon garlic powder
- Salt to taste

Preparation:

1. Preheat the oven to 400°F (200°C).
2. Pat the chickpeas dry with a paper towel.
3. In a bowl, toss chickpeas with olive oil, chili powder, cumin, garlic powder, and salt until coated.
4. Spread the chickpeas on a baking sheet in a single layer.
5. Roast in the preheated oven for 25-30 minutes, or until crispy, shaking the pan occasionally.
6. Let cool before serving.

Nutrient Facts (per serving):

- Calories: Approximately 130 per serving
- Carbohydrates: 18g
- Fat: 4g
- Protein: 6g

40. Guacamole with Veggie Sticks

Prep.Time: 5 min

Cook Time: 0 min

Serving: 1

Beverage pairing: Water

Ingredients:

- 1 ripe avocado
- 1/2 lime, juiced
- 1/4 teaspoon garlic powder
- Salt and pepper to taste
- Assorted vegetable sticks (carrots, celery, bell peppers)

Preparation:

1. In a bowl, mash the avocado with lime juice, garlic powder, salt, and pepper until smooth.
2. Serve with assorted vegetable sticks for dipping.

Nutrient Facts (per serving):

- Calories: Approximately 120 per serving
- Carbohydrates: 8g
- Fat: 10g
- Protein: 2g

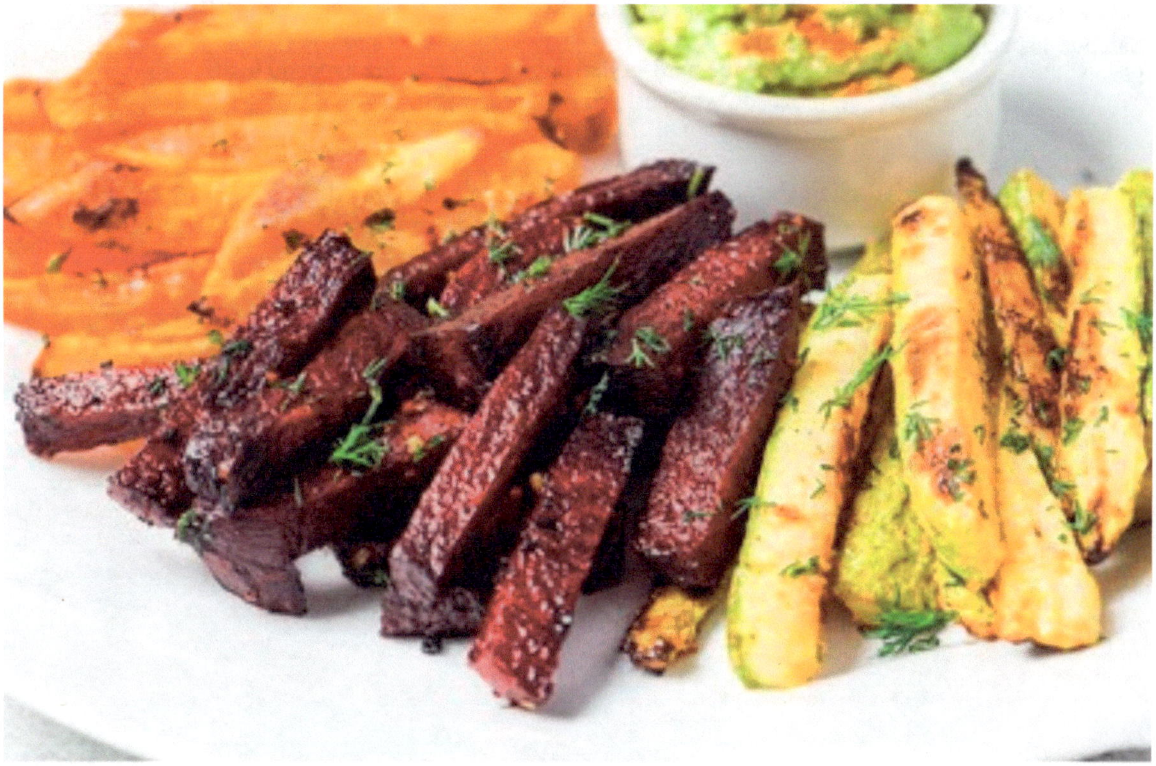

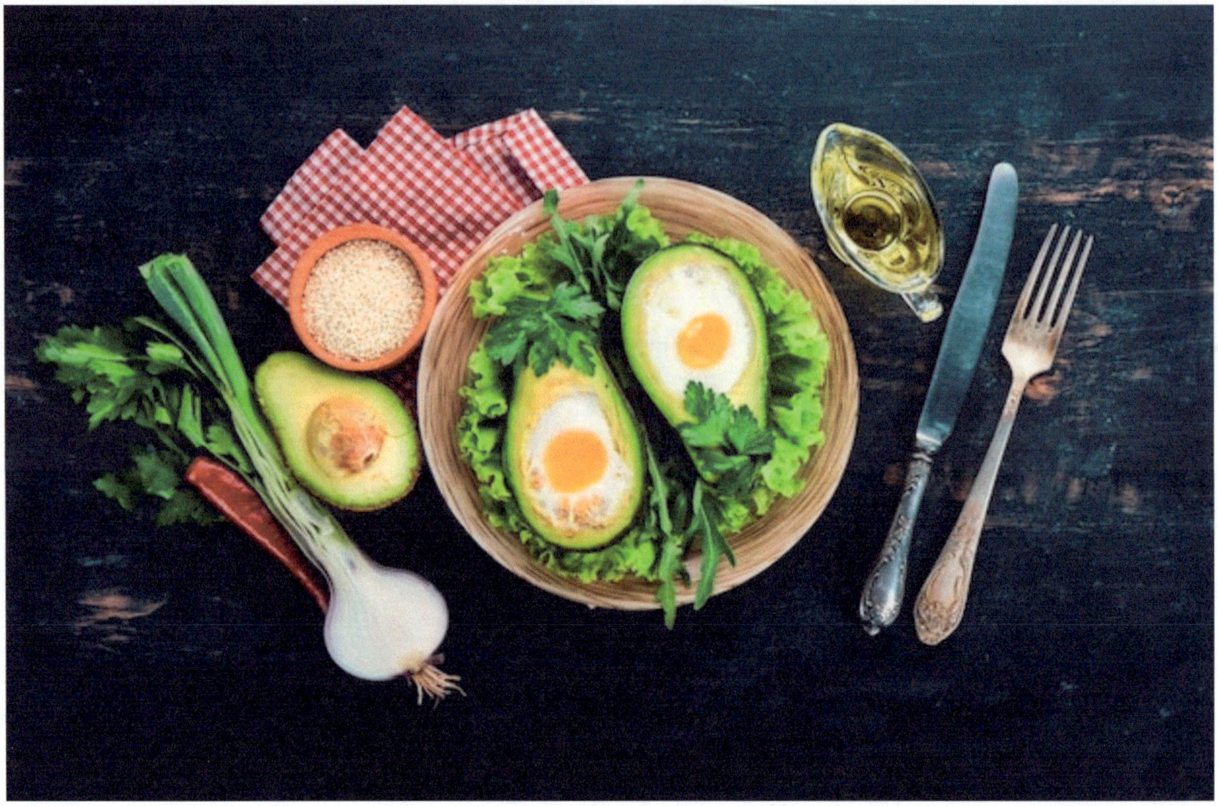

41. Hard-Boiled Egg and Avocado Boat

Prep.Time:	**Cook Time:**	**Serving:**	**Beverage pairing:**
5 min	0 min	1	Black Tea

Ingredients:

- 1 hard-boiled egg
- 1/2 avocado
- Salt and pepper to taste

Preparation:

1. Cut the hard-boiled egg in half.
2. Remove the pit from the avocado and scoop out some flesh to create a "boat."
3. Place the hard-boiled egg halves into the avocado boats.
4. Season with salt and pepper to taste.

Nutrient Facts (per serving):

- Calories: Approximately 200 per serving
- Carbohydrates: 7g
- Fat: 16g
- Protein: 10g

42. Turkey Jerky

Prep.Time: 10 min

Cook Time: 3-4 Hour

Serving: 1

Beverage pairing: Green Tea

Ingredients:

- 1 pound turkey breast, thinly sliced
- 1/4 cup soy sauce (low-sodium)
- 2 tablespoons Worcestershire sauce
- 1 tablespoon honey (optional)
- 1 teaspoon garlic powder
- 1 teaspoon onion powder
- 1/2 teaspoon black pepper
- 1/2 teaspoon smoked paprika

Preparation:

1. In a bowl, mix together soy sauce, Worcestershire sauce, honey (if using), garlic powder, onion powder, black pepper, and smoked paprika.
2. Add the turkey slices to the marinade, making sure they are fully coated. Marinate in the refrigerator for at least 1 hour or overnight.
3. Preheat the oven to 175°F (80°C) or the lowest setting.
4. Remove the turkey slices from the marinade and pat dry with paper towels.
5. Place the turkey slices on a baking sheet lined with parchment paper.
6. Bake in the preheated oven for 3-4 hours, or until the turkey is dried and firm.
7. Let cool before serving. Store in an airtight container.

Nutrient Facts (per serving):

- Calories: Approximately 100 per serving
- Carbohydrates: 0g
- Fat: 1g
- Protein: 20g

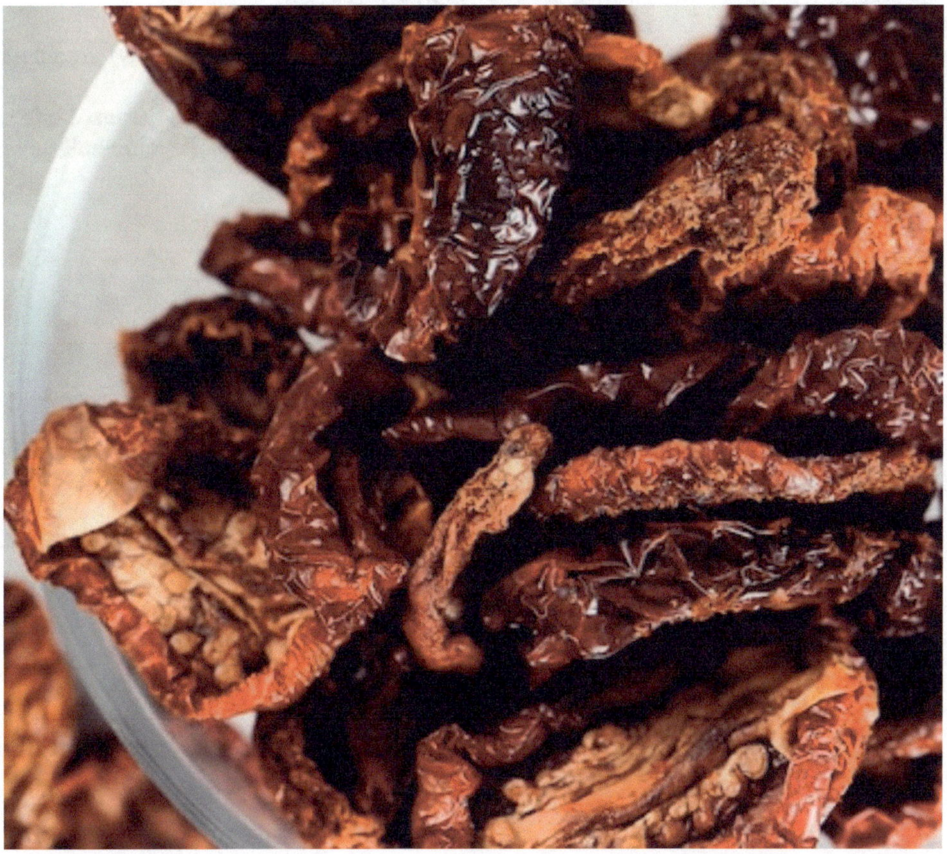

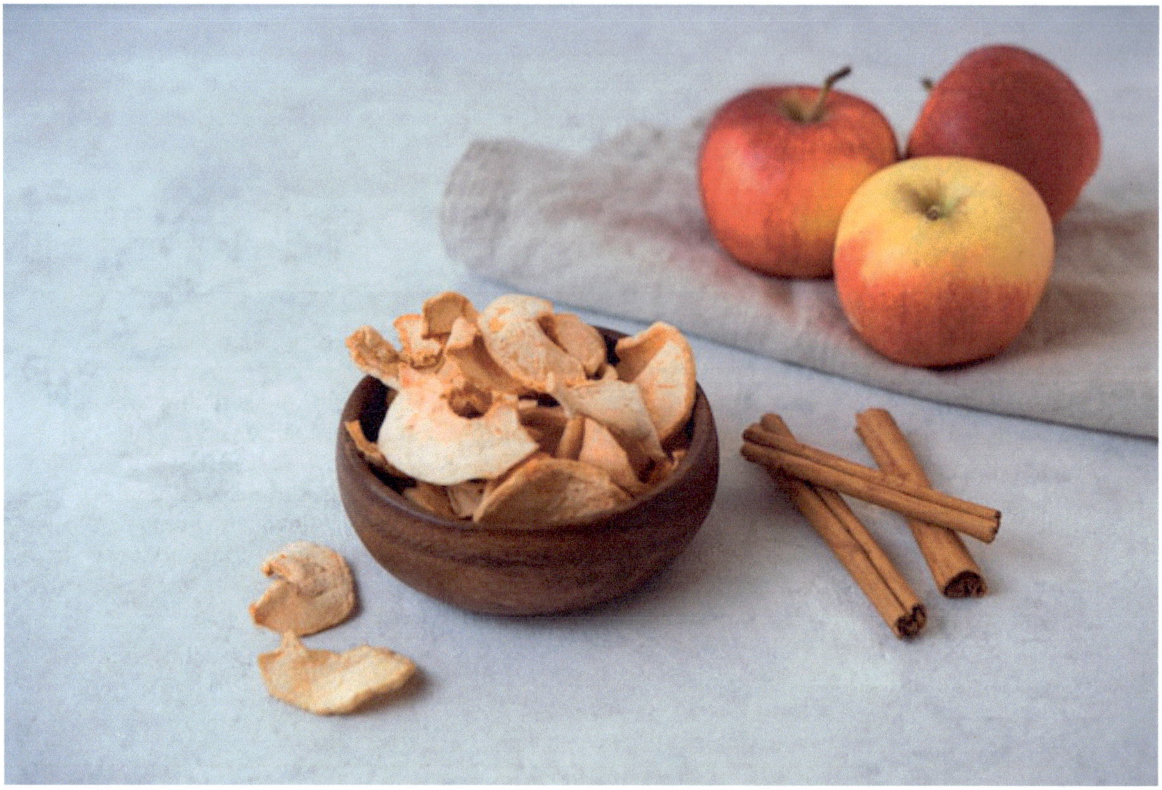

43. Cinnamon Apple Chips

Prep.Time: 10 min

Cook Time: 2-3 Hour

Serving: 1

Beverage pairing: Herbal Tea

Ingredients:

- 2 apples, cored and thinly sliced
- 1 tablespoon cinnamon
- 1 tablespoon granulated sweetener (optional)

Preparation:

1. Preheat the oven to 200°F (95°C).
2. Line a baking sheet with parchment paper.
3. In a bowl, toss the apple slices with cinnamon and granulated sweetener (if using), until evenly coated.
4. Place the apple slices in a single layer on the prepared baking sheet.
5. Bake in the preheated oven for 2-3 hours, flipping halfway through, until the apple slices are dried and crispy.
6. Let cool before serving.

Nutrient Facts (per serving):

- Calories: Approximately 50 per serving
- Carbohydrates: 13g
- Fat: 0g
- Protein: 0g

44. Caprese Salad Skewers

Prep.Time:	Cook Time:	Serving:	Beverage pairing:
10 min	0 min	1	Mint Water

Ingredients:

- Cherry tomatoes
- Fresh mozzarella balls
- Fresh basil leaves
- Balsamic glaze (optional)

Preparation:

1. Thread cherry tomatoes, fresh mozzarella balls, and fresh basil leaves onto skewers.
2. Drizzle with balsamic glaze if desired.

Nutrient Facts (per serving):

- Calories: Approximately 100 per serving
- Carbohydrates: 3g
- Fat: 8g
- Protein: 5g

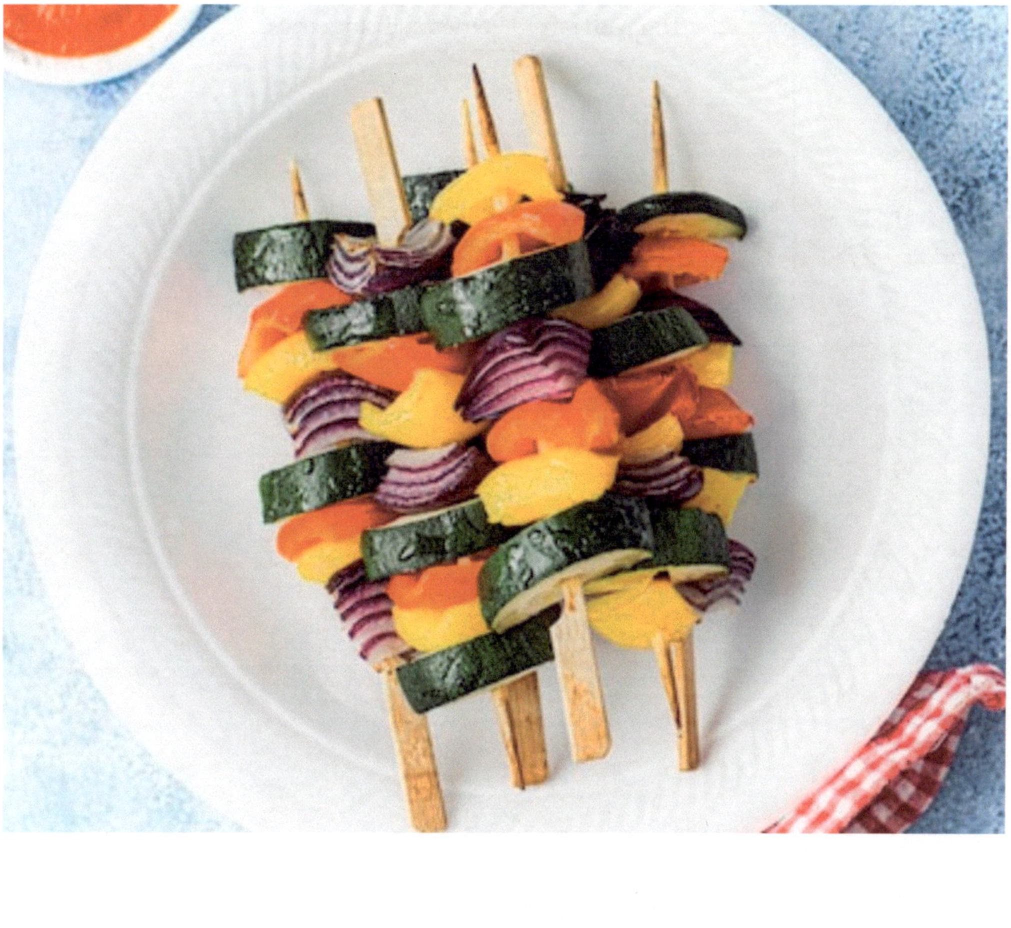

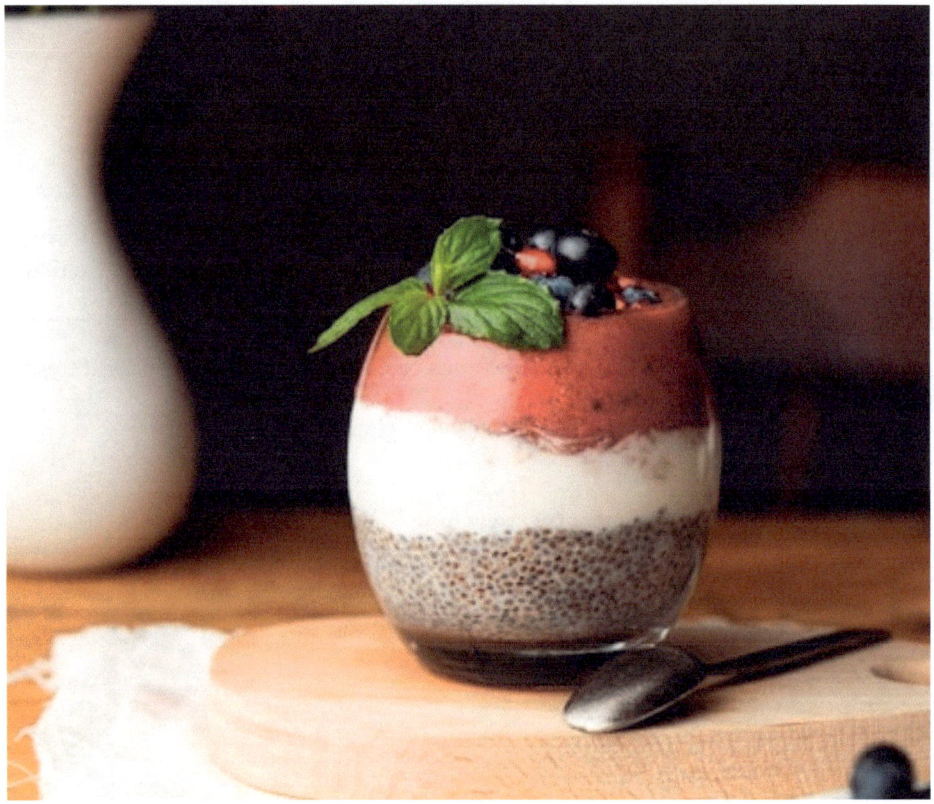

45. Greek Yogurt with Berries and Chia Seeds

Prep.Time:	Cook Time:	Serving:	Beverage pairing:
2 min	0 min	1	Water

Ingredients:

- 1/2 cup Greek yogurt (low-fat or non-fat)
- 1/4 cup mixed berries (such as strawberries, blueberries, raspberries)
- 1 tablespoon chia seeds

Preparation:

1. Spoon the Greek yogurt into a bowl.
2. Top with mixed berries and chia seeds.

Nutrient Facts (per serving):

- Calories: Approximately 150 per serving
- Carbohydrates: 15g
- Fat: 5g
- Protein: 12g

46. Roasted Brussels Sprouts with Balsamic Glaze

Prep.Time: 10 min

Cook Time: 20 min

Serving: 1

Beverage pairing: Cucumber Water

Ingredients:

- 1 pound Brussels sprouts, trimmed and halved
- 2 tablespoons olive oil
- Salt and pepper to taste
- Balsamic glaze for drizzling

Preparation:

1. Preheat the oven to 400°F (200°C).
2. In a bowl, toss Brussels sprouts with olive oil, salt, and pepper until coated.
3. Spread the Brussels sprouts on a baking sheet in a single layer.
4. Roast in the preheated oven for 20-25 minutes, or until tender and caramelized.
5. Drizzle with balsamic glaze before serving.

Nutrient Facts (per serving):

- Calories: Approximately 100 per serving
- Carbohydrates: 12g
- Fat: 5g
- Protein: 4g

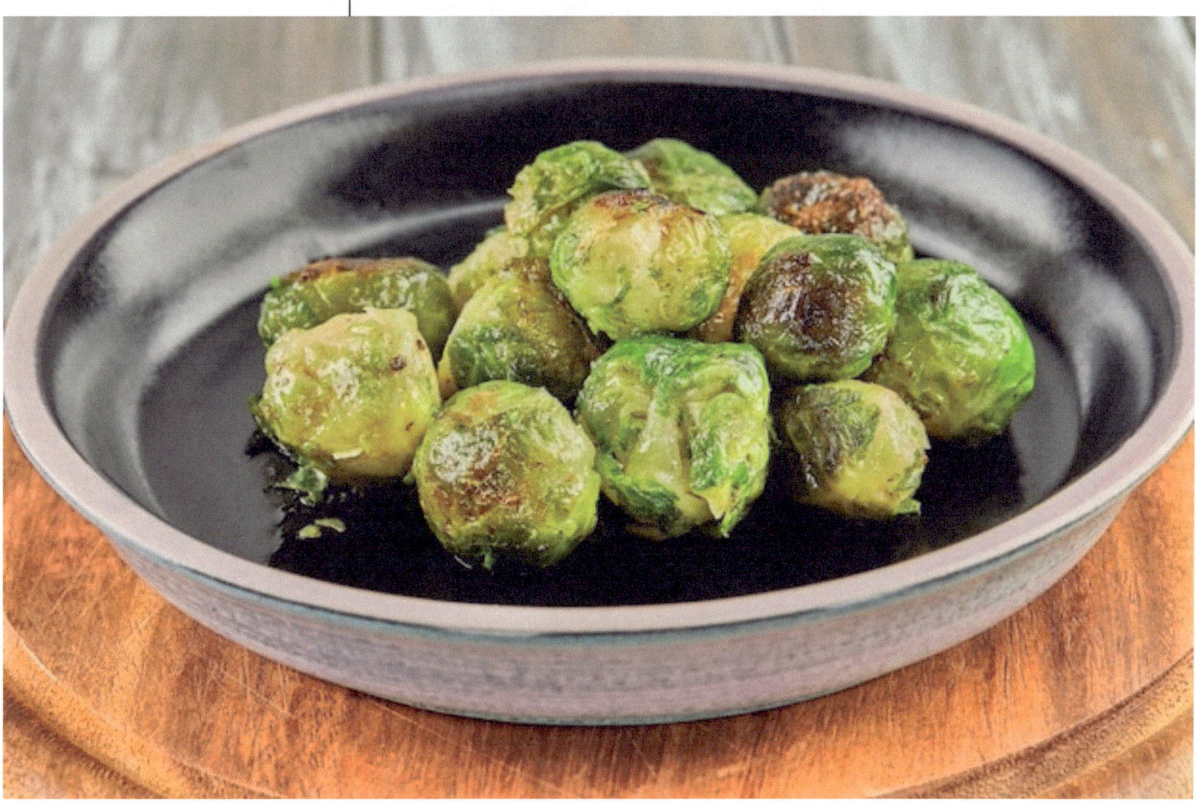

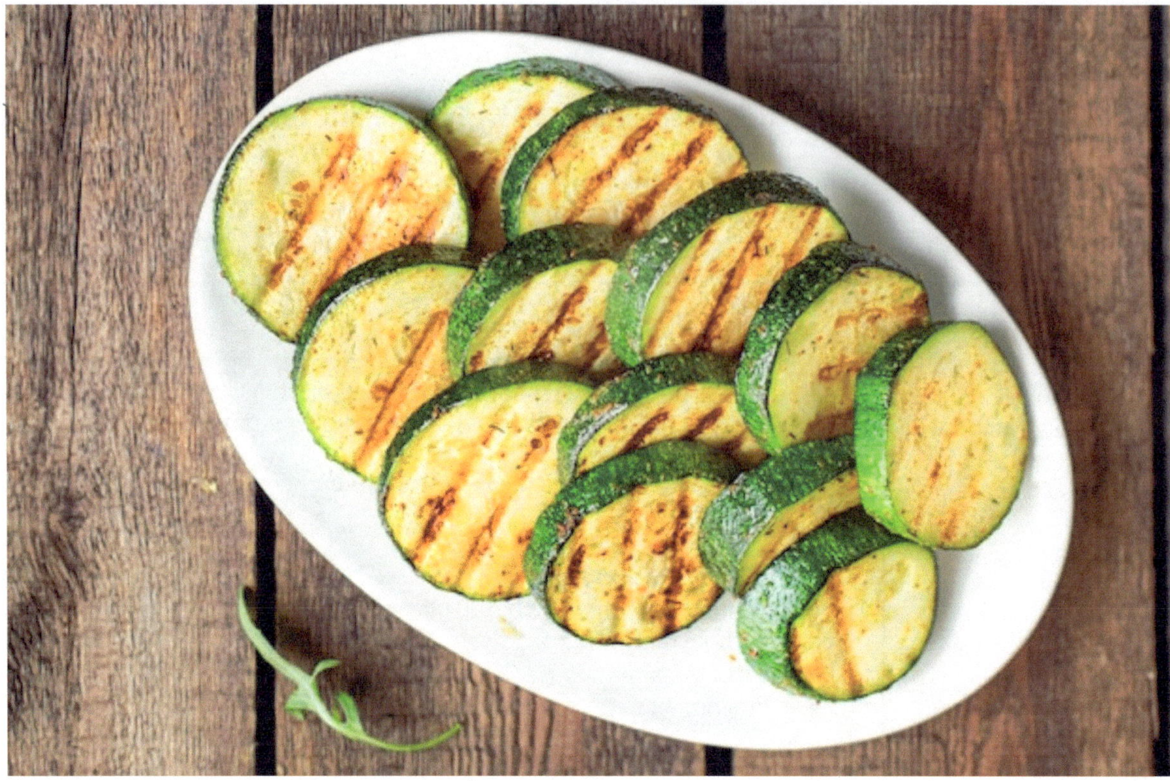

47. Baked Zucchini Chips

Prep.Time: 10 min

Cook Time: 15-20 min

Serving: 1

Beverage pairing: Black Coffee

Ingredients:

- 2 medium zucchini, thinly sliced
- 1 tablespoon olive oil
- 1/4 cup grated Parmesan cheese
- 1/2 teaspoon garlic powder
- Salt and pepper to taste

Preparation:

1. Preheat the oven to 425°F (220°C).
2. In a bowl, toss zucchini slices with olive oil, Parmesan cheese, garlic powder, salt, and pepper until evenly coated.
3. Arrange the zucchini slices on a baking sheet lined with parchment paper.
4. Bake in the preheated oven for 15-20 minutes, or until golden and crispy.
5. Let cool before serving.

Nutrient Facts (per serving):

- Calories: Approximately 80 per serving
- Carbohydrates: 7g
- Fat: 5g
- Protein: 3g

48. Peanut Butter and Banana Sandwich

Prep.Time: 5 min

Cook Time: 0 min

Serving: 1

Beverage pairing: Black Coffee

Ingredients:

- 2 slices whole grain bread (sugar-free)
- 2 tablespoons peanut butter (unsweetened)
- 1 small banana, sliced

Preparation:

1. Spread peanut butter evenly on one slice of bread.
2. Arrange banana slices on top of the peanut butter.
3. Place the second slice of bread on top to form a sandwich.
4. Cut the sandwich in half if desired.

Nutrient Facts (per serving):

- Calories: Approximately 300 per serving
- Carbohydrates: 35g
- Fat: 15g
- Protein: 8g

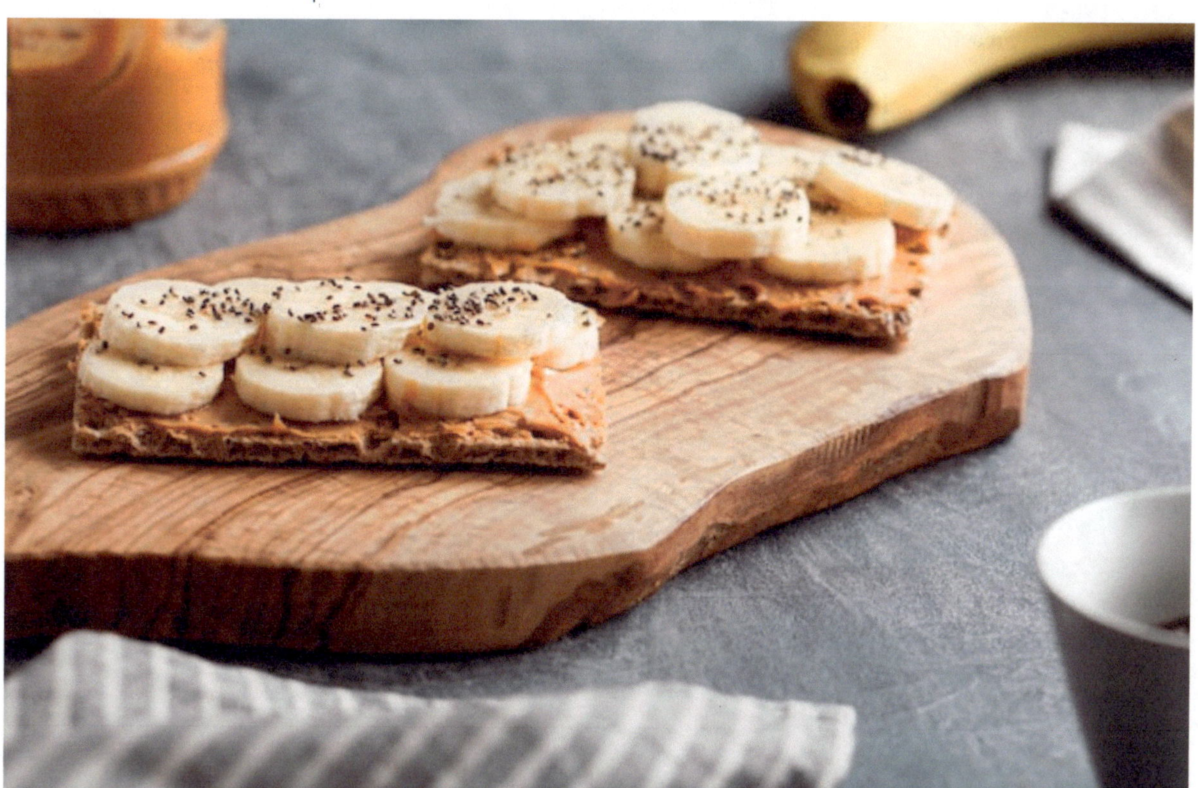

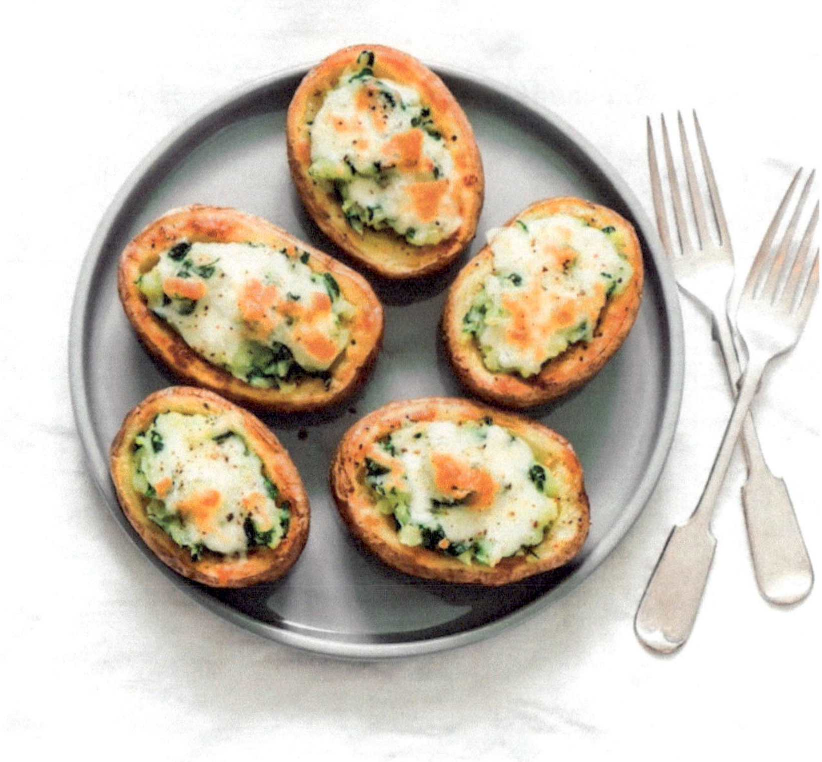

49. Mini Frittatas with Spinach and Feta

Prep.Time:	Cook Time:	Serving:	Beverage pairing:
10 min	12-15 min	1	Water

Ingredients:

- 4 eggs
- 1/4 cup spinach, chopped
- 2 tablespoons crumbled feta cheese
- Salt and pepper to taste

Preparation:

1. Preheat the oven to 350°F (175°C).
2. In a bowl, beat the eggs until well mixed.
3. Stir in chopped spinach and crumbled feta cheese. Season with salt and pepper.
4. Grease a mini muffin tin and pour the egg mixture evenly into each cup.
5. Bake in the preheated oven for 12-15 minutes, or until set.
6. Let cool slightly before removing from the muffin tin.

Nutrient Facts (per serving):

- Calories: Approximately 100 per serving
- Carbohydrates: 2g
- Fat: 7g
- Protein: 8g

50. Sugar-Free Chocolate Covered Strawberries

Prep.Time:	Cook Time:	Serving:	Beverage pairing:
15 min	0 min	1	Black Coffee

Ingredients:

- Fresh strawberries
- Sugar-free chocolate chips
- 1 teaspoon coconut oil (optional)

Preparation:

1. Wash and dry the strawberries, leaving the stems intact.
2. In a microwave-safe bowl, melt the sugar-free chocolate chips with coconut oil (if using), stirring until smooth.
3. Dip each strawberry into the melted chocolate, coating evenly.
4. Place the chocolate-covered strawberries on a parchment-lined tray.
5. Refrigerate for 10-15 minutes, or until the chocolate sets.

Nutrient Facts (per serving):

- Calories: Approximately 50 per serving
- Carbohydrates: 8g
- Fat: 3g
- Protein: 1g

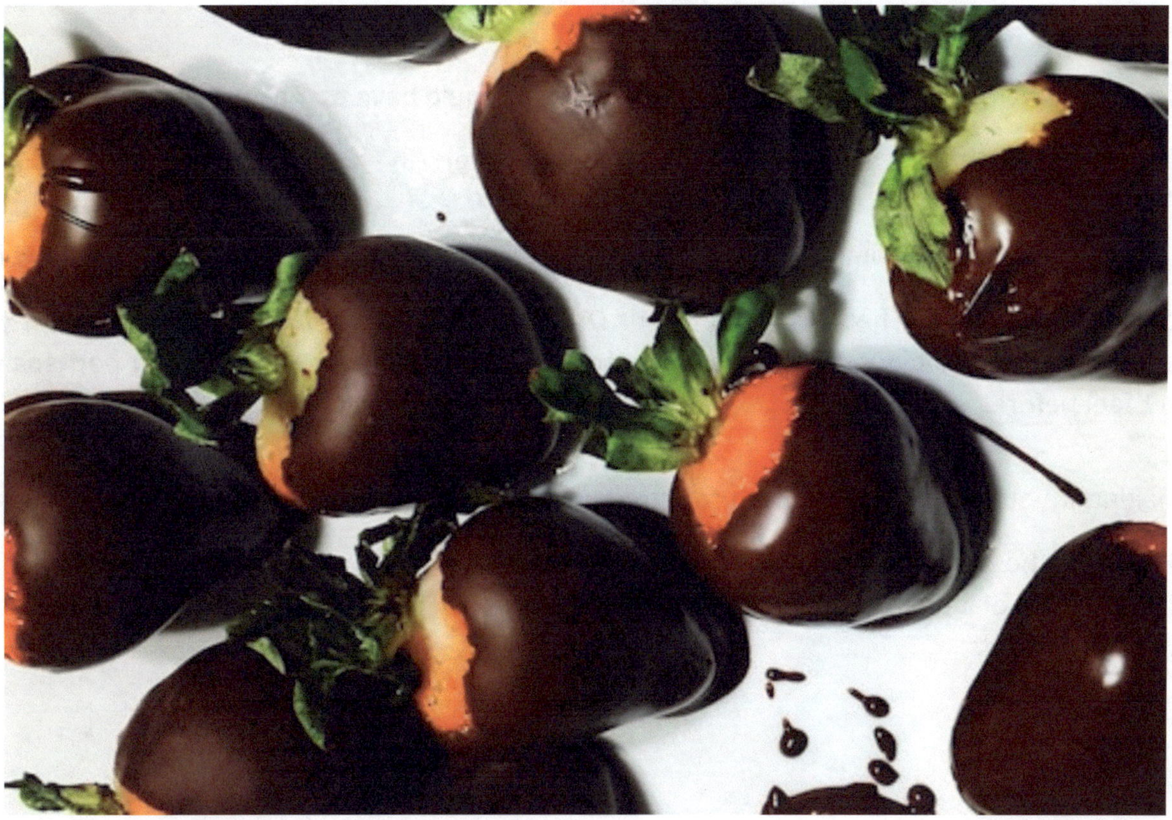

Your Kindness is Key

Share Your Experience, Share Your Strength

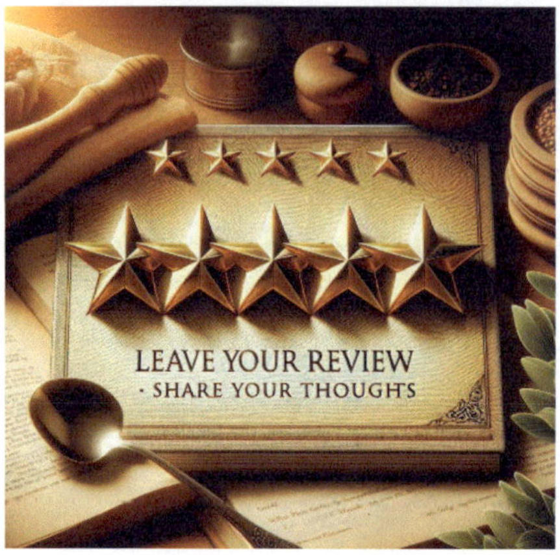

"Helping one person might not change the whole world, but it could change the world for one person." - Anonymous

---

Do you remember what it was like when you first heard the words "Type 2 Diabetes?" Perhaps it felt like a mountain you weren't sure you could climb.

Maybe it was daunting, thinking about the changes you'd have to make in your life, especially with your diet. It's a journey many embark on feeling uncertain and alone.

But you've found a companion on this journey, haven't you? Type 2 Diabetes Cookbook Beginner's Quick & Easy Recipes for Delicious Diabetes Diets by Lily Anders has been with you, offering guidance, delicious recipes, and a sense of control over your diabetes that perhaps you didn't feel before.

Imagine if you could light the path for someone just starting on this journey. Someone who feels lost in the sea of information, unsure of where to turn for reliable, practical advice on managing their diabetes through diet. Your experience, shared through a review, could be the beacon they need.

This isn't just about leaving a review; it's about extending a hand, offering support, and sharing the strength that comes from knowledge and community. Your words could help another person find their footing, making their journey a bit easier and less lonely.

So, here's my humble request on behalf of a fellow journeyer you've yet to meet:

Please take a moment to share your experience with the book. Your insights could be the very thing another person needs to hear to take that first, brave step toward a healthier, happier life with diabetes. Your review, a simple act of kindness, asks for nothing in return yet offers immeasurable value.

To leave your review, just follow this link:

https://www.amazon.com/review/create-review/?ie=UTF8&channel=glance-detail&asin=1963939360

If the thought of helping another soul on their diabetes journey warms your heart, then you're exactly who I hoped to reach with this book. Welcome to a community where kindness, support, and shared victories pave the way to a better life.

I'm beyond grateful for your help in spreading the word and even more excited to continue providing you with the knowledge and recipes to make managing diabetes not just manageable, but enjoyable.

Click the QR Code Here!

Thank you from the deepest places in my heart. Your generosity makes all the difference.

Lily Anders

P.S. - Sharing is caring, they say. If you believe this book has brought value to your life and could do the same for someone else, consider sharing it with them. It's another beautiful way to change a life, one meal at a time.

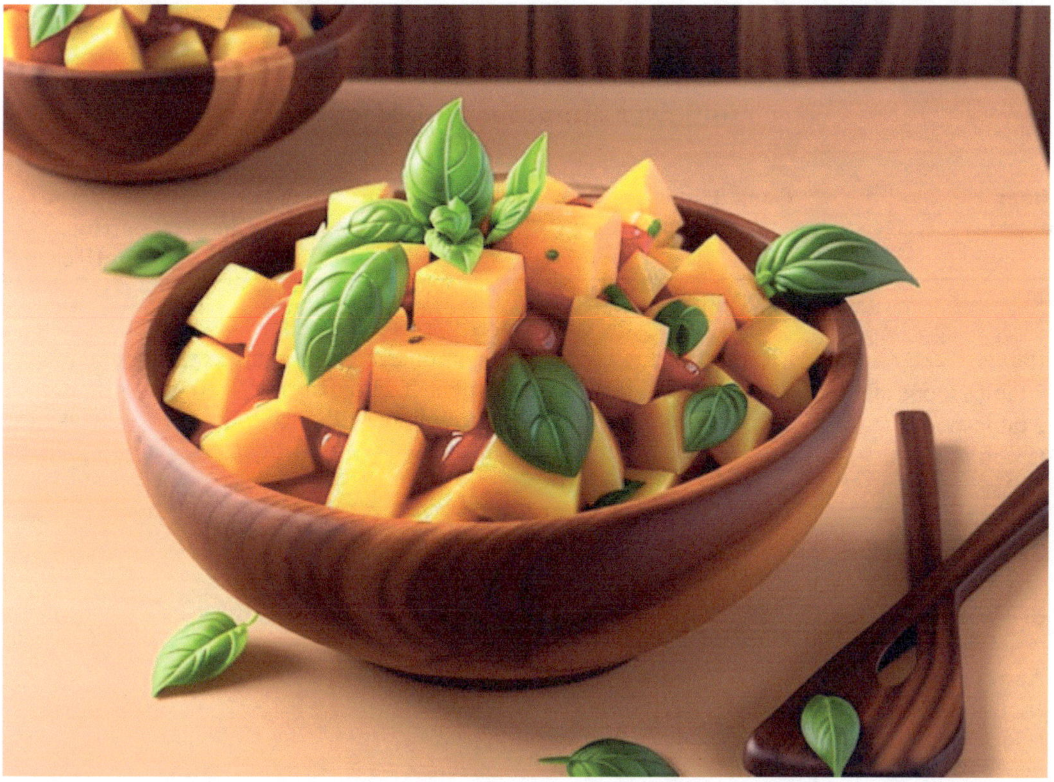

51. Cubed Mango with Tajin Seasoning

Prep.Time: 5 min	Cook Time: 0 min	Serving: 1	Beverage pairing: Lemonade

Ingredients:

- 1 ripe mango, cubed
- Tajin seasoning (chili powder, lime, salt)

Preparation:

1. Arrange mango cubes on a plate.
2. Sprinkle Tajin seasoning over the mango slices to taste.

Nutrient Facts (per serving):

- Calories: Approximately 80 per serving
- Carbohydrates: 20g
- Fat: 0g
- Protein: 1g

52. Cauliflower Hummus with Veggie Dippers

Prep.Time: 15 min | **Cook Time:** 10 min | **Serving:** 1 | **Beverage pairing:** Mint Tea

Ingredients:

- 2 cups cauliflower florets
- 2 tablespoons tahini
- 2 tablespoons lemon juice
- 1 clove garlic, minced
- 2 tablespoons olive oil
- Salt and pepper to taste
- Assorted vegetable sticks (carrots, celery, bell peppers)

Preparation:

1. Steam the cauliflower florets until tender.
2. In a food processor, combine steamed cauliflower, tahini, lemon juice, minced garlic, olive oil, salt, and pepper. Blend until smooth.
3. Serve the cauliflower hummus with assorted vegetable sticks for dipping.

Nutrient Facts (per serving):

- Calories: Approximately 80 per serving
- Carbohydrates: 6g
- Fat: 5g
- Protein: 3g

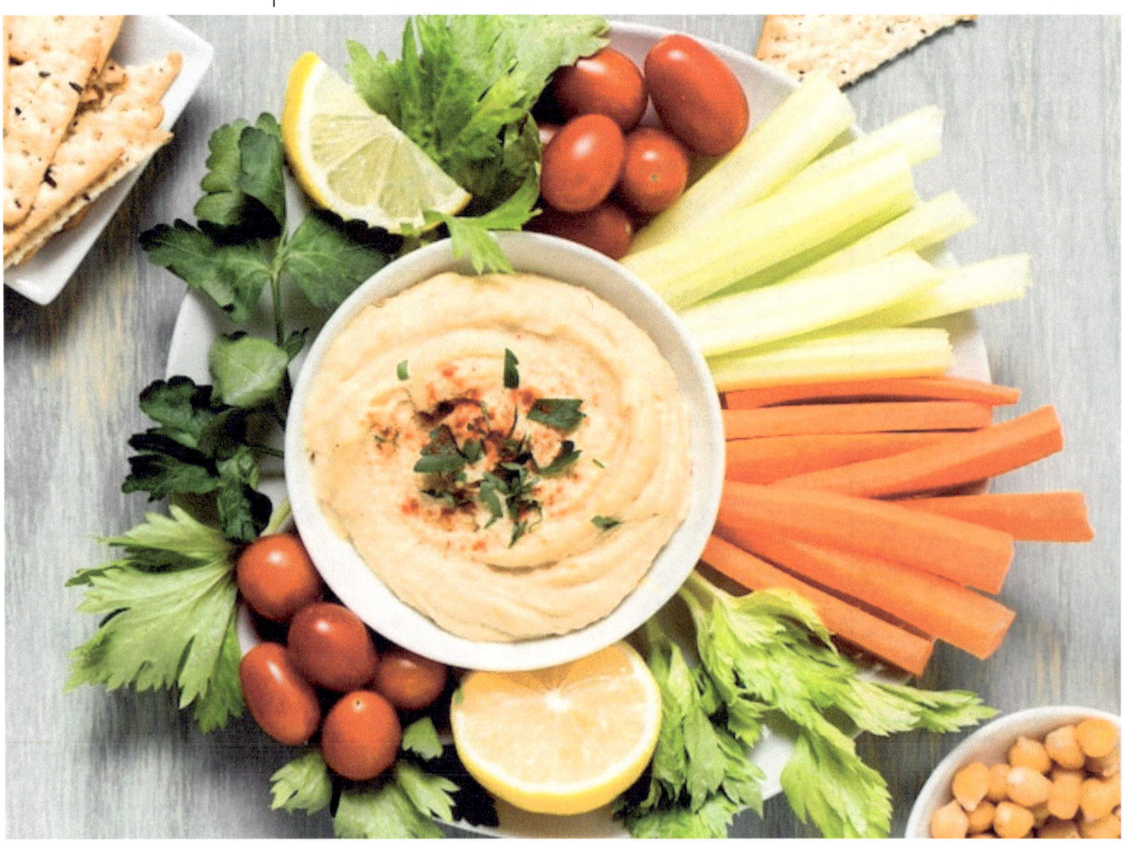

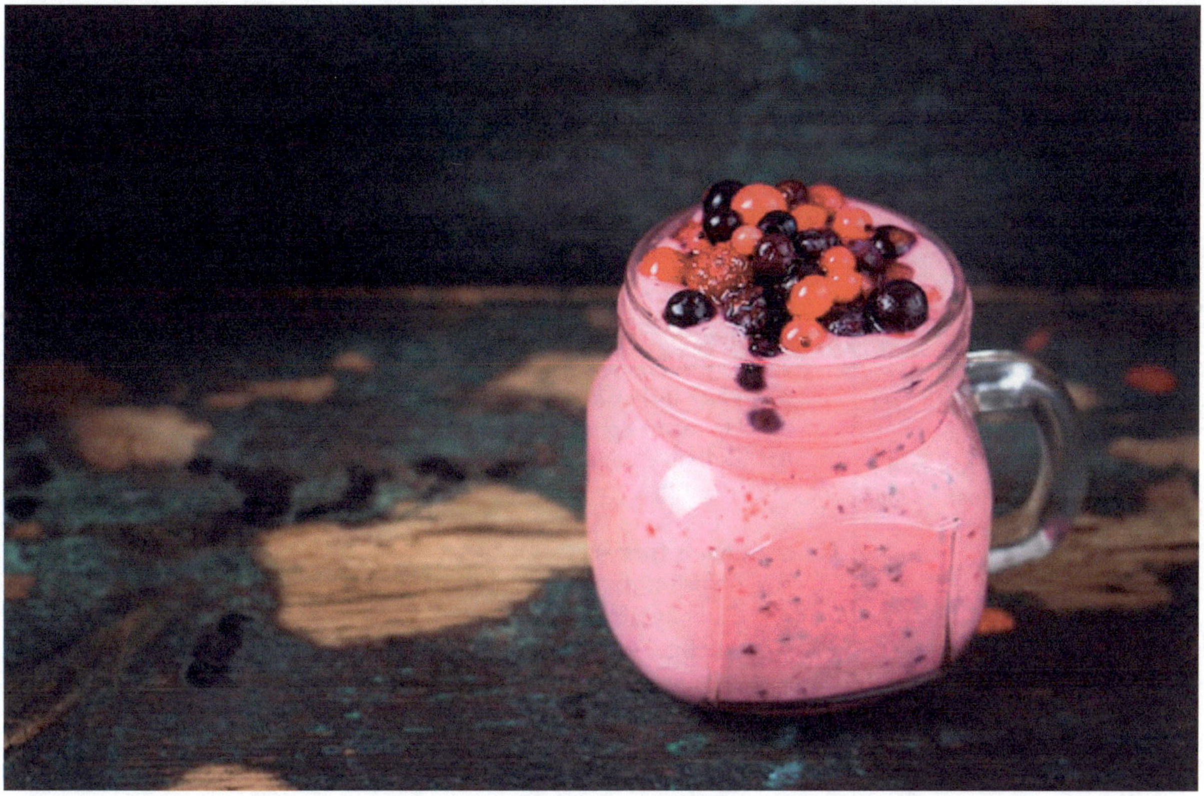

53. Berry Blast Smoothie

Prep.Time: 5 min | **Cook Time:** 0 min | **Serving:** 1 | **Beverage pairing:** Iced Tea

Ingredients:

- 1 cup mixed berries (such as strawberries, blueberries, and raspberries)
- 1/2 banana
- 1/2 cup plain Greek yogurt
- 1/2 cup almond milk (or any milk of your choice)
- 1 tablespoon honey or maple syrup (optional)
- Ice cubes (optional)

Preparation:

1. In a blender, combine mixed berries, banana, Greek yogurt, almond milk, and honey or maple syrup if using.
2. Blend until smooth and creamy. If desired, add ice cubes and blend again until smooth.
3. Pour the smoothie into glasses and serve immediately.
4. Enjoy this refreshing Berry Blast Smoothie as a nutritious snack or breakfast option.

Nutrient Facts (per serving):

- Calories: Approximately 150 per serving
- Carbohydrates: 25g
- Fat: 2g
- Protein: 5g

54. Turkey and Avocado Lettuce Wraps

Prep.Time:	Cook Time:	Serving:	Beverage pairing:
5 min	0 min	1	Mint Water

Ingredients:

- Lettuce leaves
- Sliced turkey breast
- Avocado slices
- Optional: Mustard or mayonnaise (sugar-free)

Preparation:

1. Lay out lettuce leaves on a clean surface.
2. Place turkey slices and avocado slices on each lettuce leaf.
3. Optional: Spread mustard or mayonnaise on the turkey slices.
4. Roll up the lettuce leaves to form wraps.

Nutrient Facts (per serving):

- Calories: Approximately 150 per serving
- Carbohydrates: 5g
- Fat: 8g
- Protein: 15g

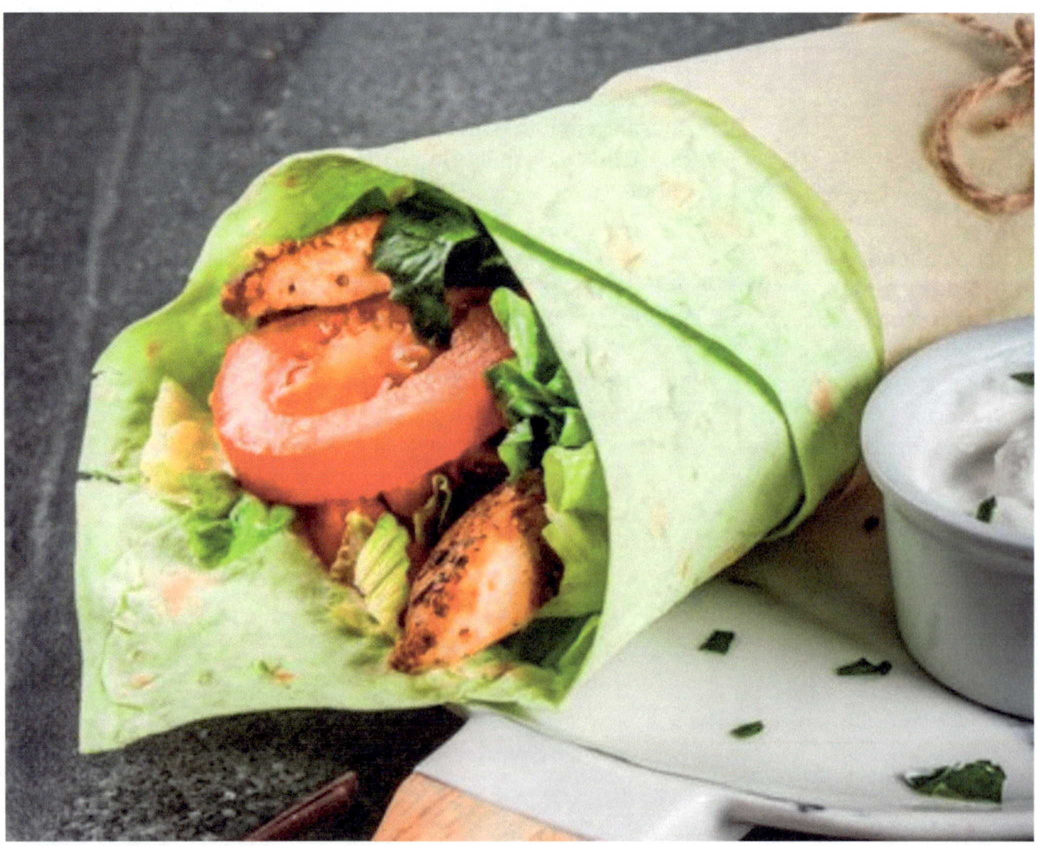

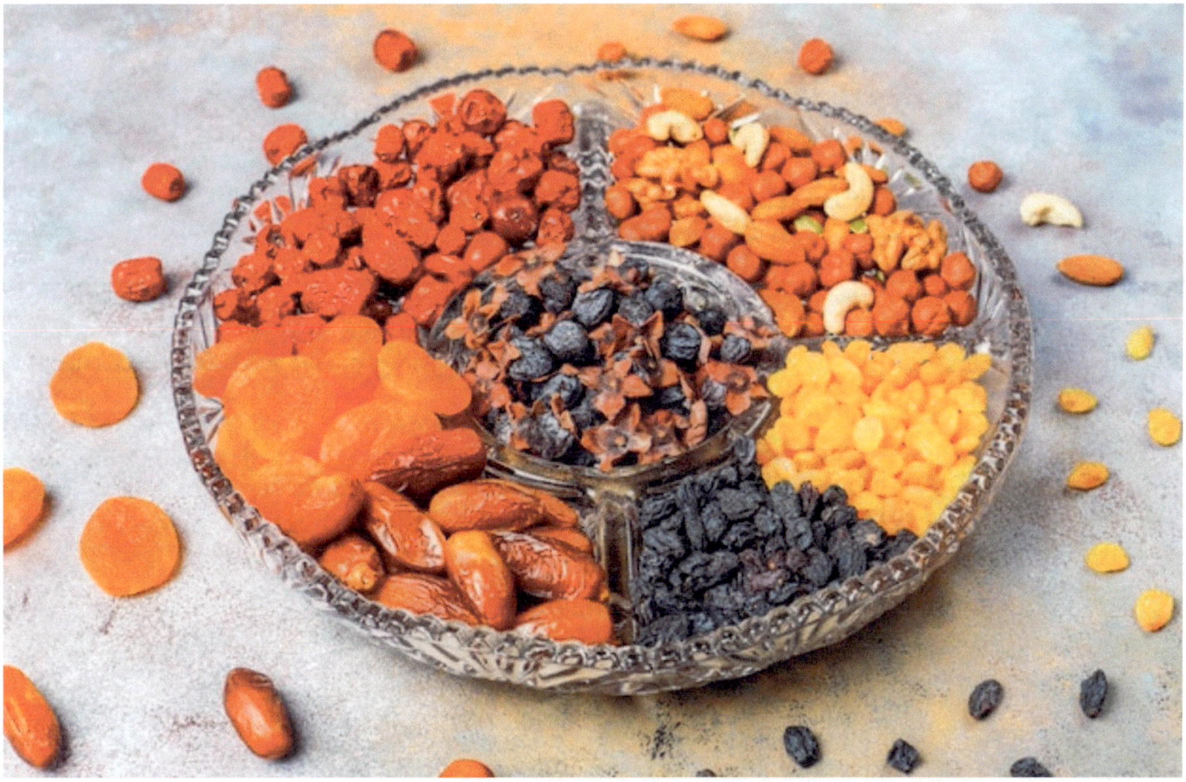

55. Seeds and Dried Fruit Mix

Prep.Time: 2 min	**Cook Time:** 0 min	**Serving:** 1	**Beverage pairing:** Black Coffee

Ingredients:

- 2 tablespoons mixed seeds (such as pumpkin seeds, sunflower seeds)
- 2 tablespoons dried fruit (such as raisins, cranberries)

Preparation:

1. Mix together seeds and dried fruit in a bowl.
2. Serve as a snack.

Nutrient Facts (per serving):

- Calories: Approximately 120 per serving
- Carbohydrates: 15g
- Fat: 6g
- Protein: 3g

56. Cucumber Cups with Tuna Salad

Prep.Time:	Cook Time:	Serving:	Beverage pairing:
15 min	0 min	1	Water

Ingredients:

- 1 large cucumber
- 1 can (5 ounces) tuna, drained
- 2 tablespoons mayonnaise (preferably sugar-free)
- 1 tablespoon diced red onion
- 1 tablespoon diced celery
- Salt and pepper to taste
- Optional: Fresh herbs for garnish

Preparation:

1. Peel the cucumber and slice it into thick rounds.
2. Use a melon baller or spoon to scoop out the seeds from each cucumber round, creating a cup.
3. In a bowl, mix together tuna, mayonnaise, diced red onion, and diced celery. Season with salt and pepper.
4. Spoon the tuna salad into each cucumber cup.
5. Garnish with fresh herbs if desired.

Nutrient Facts (per serving):

- Calories: Approximately 150 per serving
- Carbohydrates: 5g
- Fat: 8g
- Protein: 15g

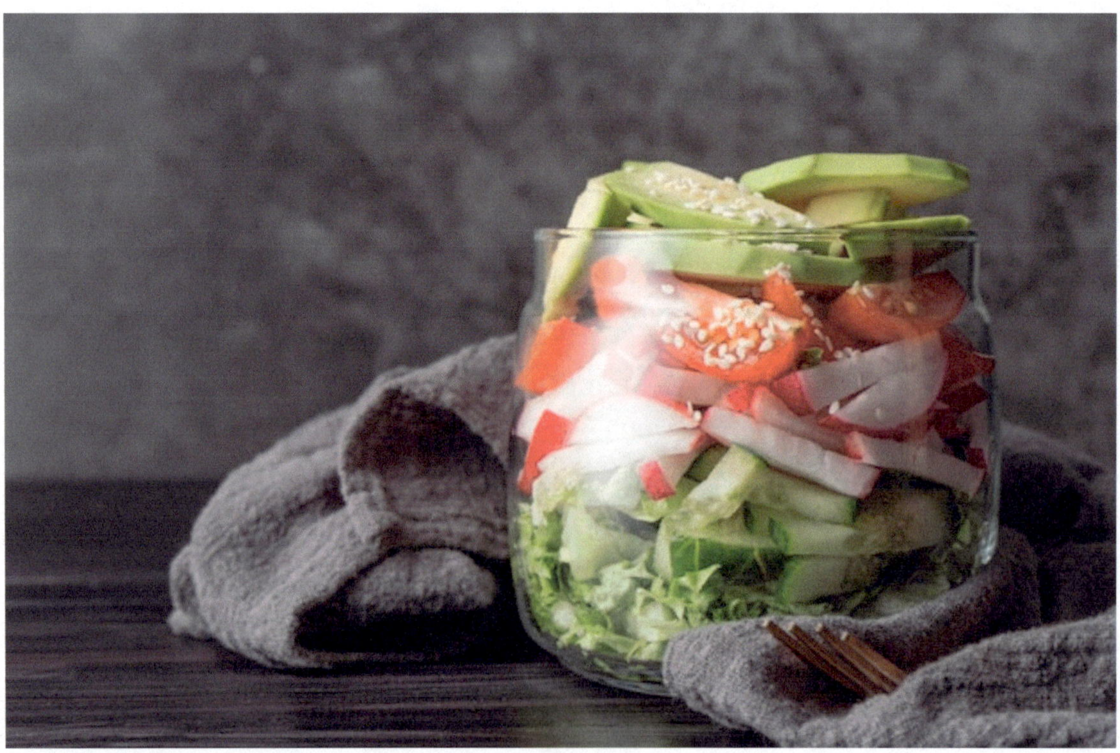

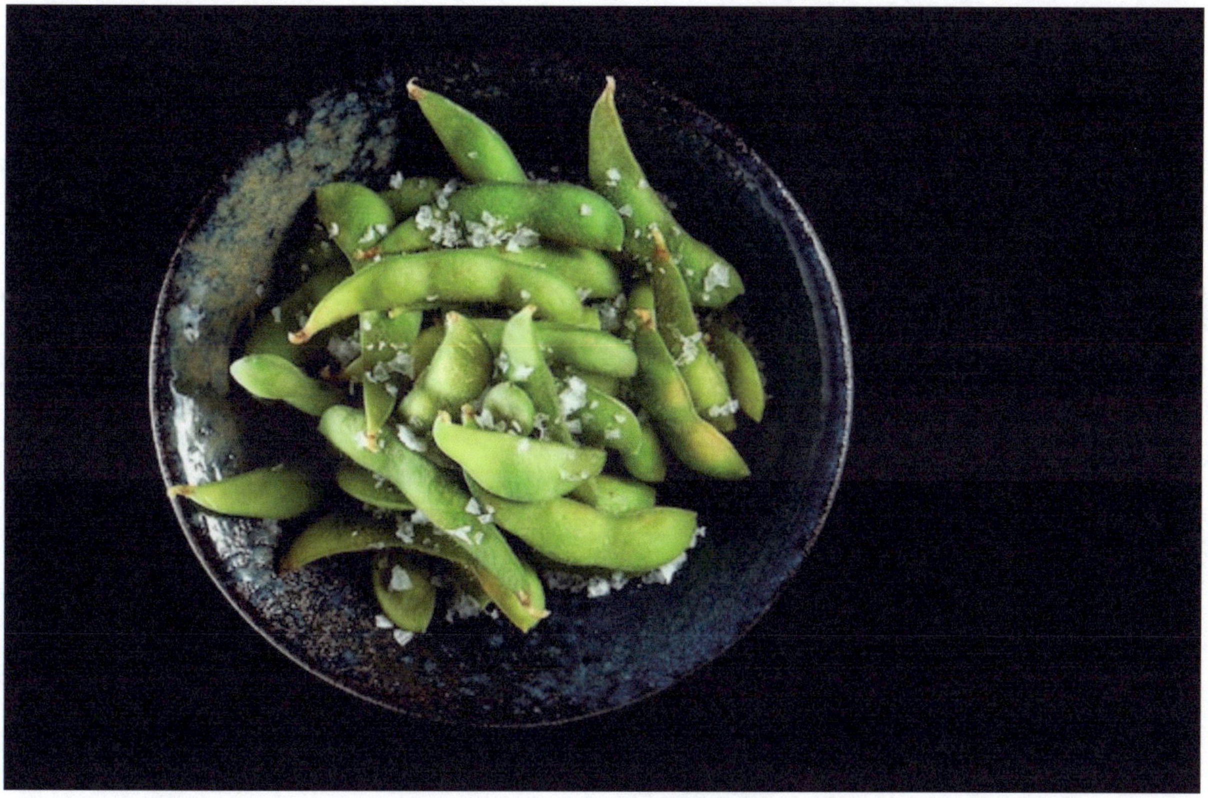

57. Roasted Edamame with Sea Salt

Prep.Time: 5 min

Cook Time: 15-20 min

Serving: 1

Beverage pairing: Black Coffee

Ingredients:

- 2 cups frozen edamame, thawed
- 1 tablespoon olive oil
- Sea salt to taste

Preparation:

1. Preheat the oven to 400°F (200°C).
2. In a bowl, toss the thawed edamame with olive oil until coated.
3. Spread the edamame on a baking sheet in a single layer.
4. Sprinkle with sea salt to taste.
5. Roast in the preheated oven for 15-20 minutes, or until crispy.
6. Let cool slightly before serving.

Nutrient Facts (per serving):

- Calories: Approximately 100 per serving
- Carbohydrates: 8g
- Fat: 3g
- Protein: 9g

58. Baked Parmesan Zucchini Sticks

Prep.Time:	Cook Time:	Serving:	Beverage pairing:
10 min	15 min	1	Herbal Tea

Ingredients:

- 2 medium zucchini
- 1/4 cup grated Parmesan cheese
- 1/4 teaspoon garlic powder
- 1/4 teaspoon dried oregano
- Salt and pepper to taste
- Cooking spray

Preparation:

1. Preheat the oven to 425°F (220°C).
2. Cut the zucchini into sticks, similar to the size of fries.
3. In a bowl, mix together grated Parmesan cheese, garlic powder, dried oregano, salt, and pepper.
4. Toss the zucchini sticks in the Parmesan mixture until evenly coated.
5. Place the coated zucchini sticks on a baking sheet lined with parchment paper.
6. Lightly spray the zucchini sticks with cooking spray.
7. Bake in the preheated oven for 15-20 minutes, or until golden and crispy.
8. Let cool slightly before serving.

Nutrient Facts (per serving):

- Calories: Approximately 100 per serving
- Carbohydrates: 5g
- Fat: 7g
- Protein: 5g

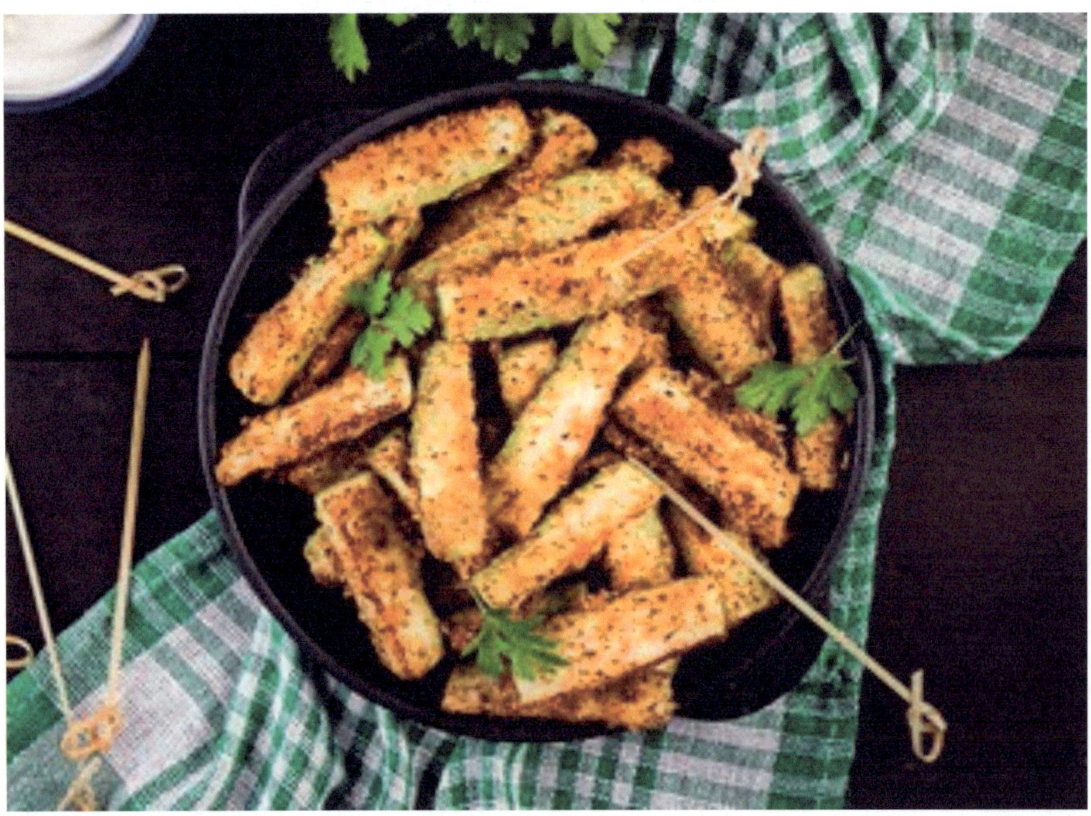

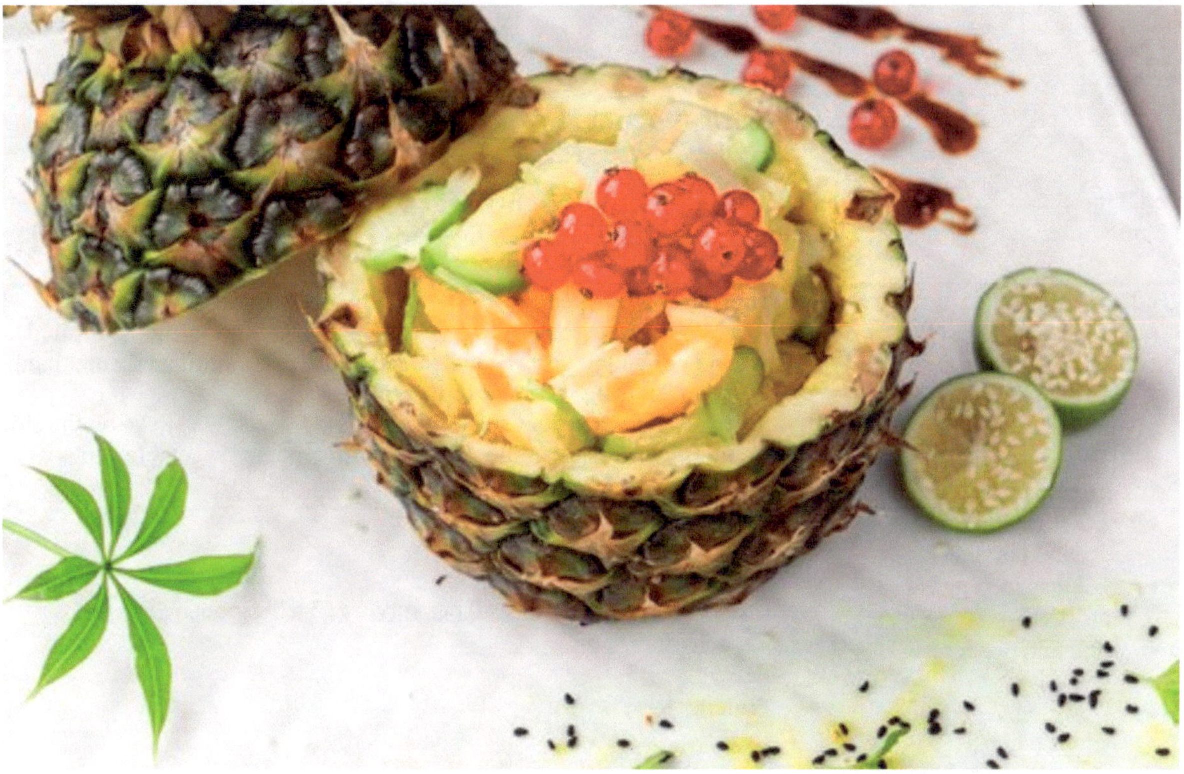

59. Cottage Cheese with Pineapple and Flaxseeds

Prep.Time:	Cook Time:	Serving:	Beverage pairing:
5 min	0 min	1	Coconut Water

Ingredients:

- 1/2 cup cottage cheese (low-fat or non-fat)
- 1/2 cup fresh pineapple chunks
- 1 tablespoon ground flaxseeds

Preparation:

1. Spoon the cottage cheese into a bowl.
2. Top with fresh pineapple chunks and ground flaxseeds.

Nutrient Facts (per serving):

- Calories: Approximately 150 per serving
- Carbohydrates: 15g
- Fat: 5g
- Protein: 12g

60. Turmeric Yogurt Dip with Veggie Sticks

Prep.Time: 5 min

Cook Time: 0 min

Serving: 1

Beverage pairing: Lemonade

Ingredients:

- 1 cup plain Greek yogurt
- 1 teaspoon ground turmeric
- 1/2 teaspoon ground cumin
- 1/2 teaspoon ground coriander
- 1/2 teaspoon garlic powder
- Salt and pepper to taste
- Assorted vegetable sticks (such as carrots, cucumbers, and bell peppers)

Preparation:

1. In a bowl, mix together plain Greek yogurt, ground turmeric, ground cumin, ground coriander, garlic powder, salt, and pepper until well combined.
2. Taste and adjust seasoning if necessary.
3. Serve the turmeric yogurt dip with assorted vegetable sticks on the side.
4. Enjoy this flavorful and healthy dip with crunchy vegetable sticks as a satisfying snack.

Nutrient Facts (per serving):

- Calories: Approximately 80 per serving (2 tablespoons dip)
- Carbohydrates: 6g
- Fat: 5g
- Protein: 3g

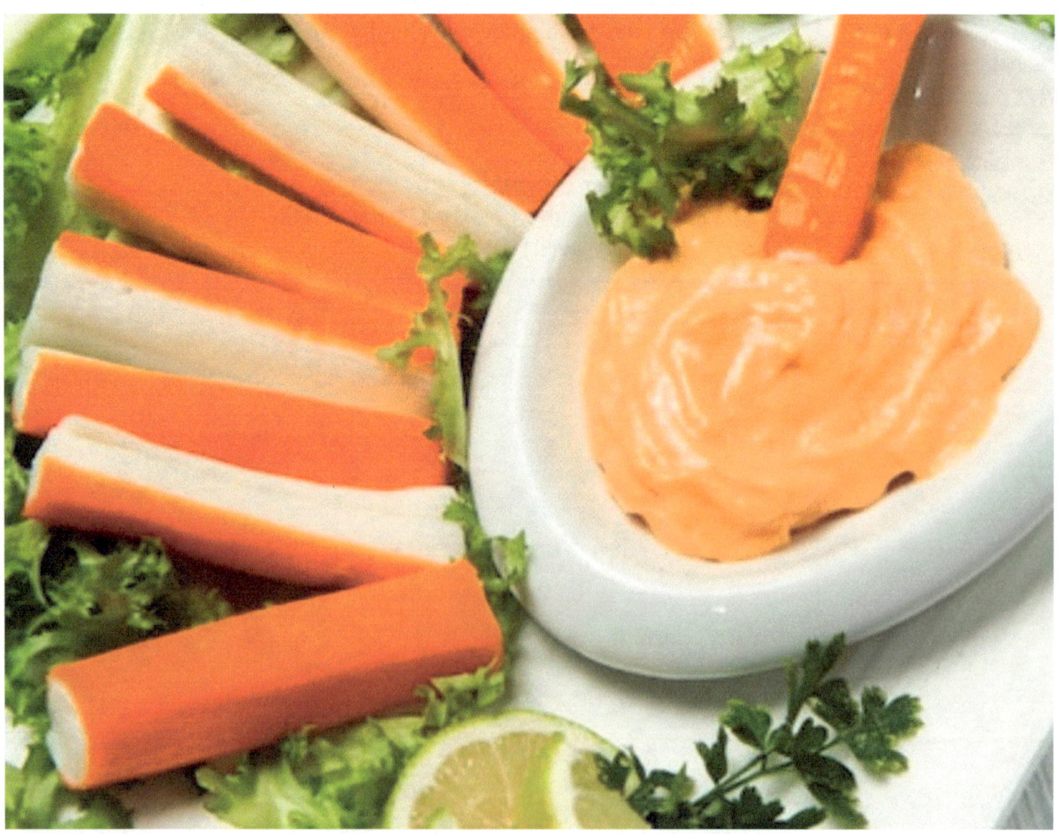

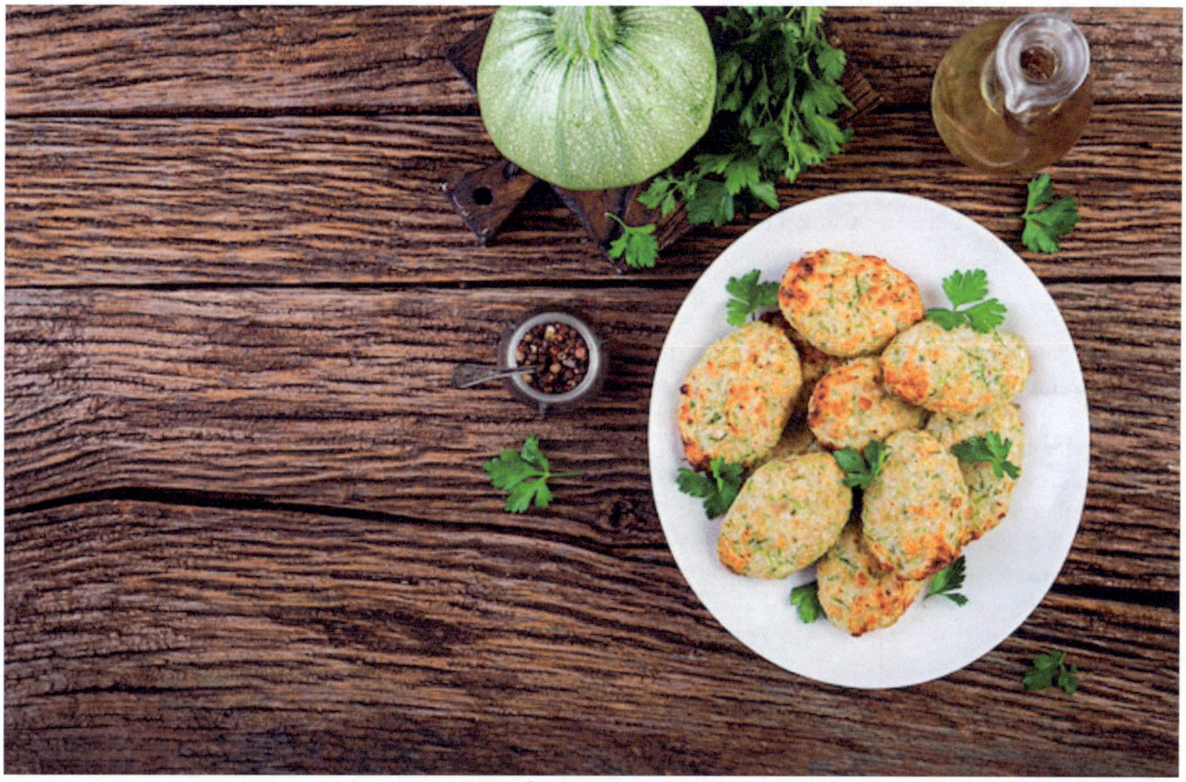

61. Broccoli and Cheddar Cheese Bites

Prep.Time: 15 min

Cook Time: 20-25 min

Serving: 1

Beverage pairing: Black Coffee

Ingredients:

- 2 cups broccoli florets, steamed and chopped
- 1/2 cup shredded cheddar cheese
- 2 eggs
- 1/4 cup almond flour
- 1/4 teaspoon garlic powder
- Salt and pepper to taste

Preparation:

1. Preheat the oven to 375°F (190°C). Grease a mini muffin tin.
2. In a bowl, mix together chopped broccoli, shredded cheddar cheese, eggs, almond flour, garlic powder, salt, and pepper until well combined.
3. Spoon the mixture into the prepared muffin tin, filling each cup almost to the top.
4. Bake in the preheated oven for 20-25 minutes, or until set and golden brown.
5. Let cool slightly before removing from the muffin tin.

Nutrient Facts (per serving):

- Calories: Approximately 100 per serving
- Carbohydrates: 5g
- Fat: 7g
- Protein: 5g

62. Trail Mix with Dark Chocolate and Almonds

Prep.Time: 2 min

Cook Time: 0 min

Serving: 1

Beverage pairing: Herbal Tea

Ingredients:

- 1/4 cup almonds
- 1/4 cup dark chocolate chips (sugar-free)
- 2 tablespoons dried cranberries (unsweetened)
- 2 tablespoons pumpkin seeds
- 2 tablespoons sunflower seeds

Preparation:

1. In a bowl, mix together almonds, dark chocolate chips, dried cranberries, pumpkin seeds, and sunflower seeds.
2. Store in an airtight container for a convenient snack on the go.

Nutrient Facts (per serving):

- Calories: Approximately 150 per serving
- Carbohydrates: 10g
- Fat: 11g
- Protein: 4g

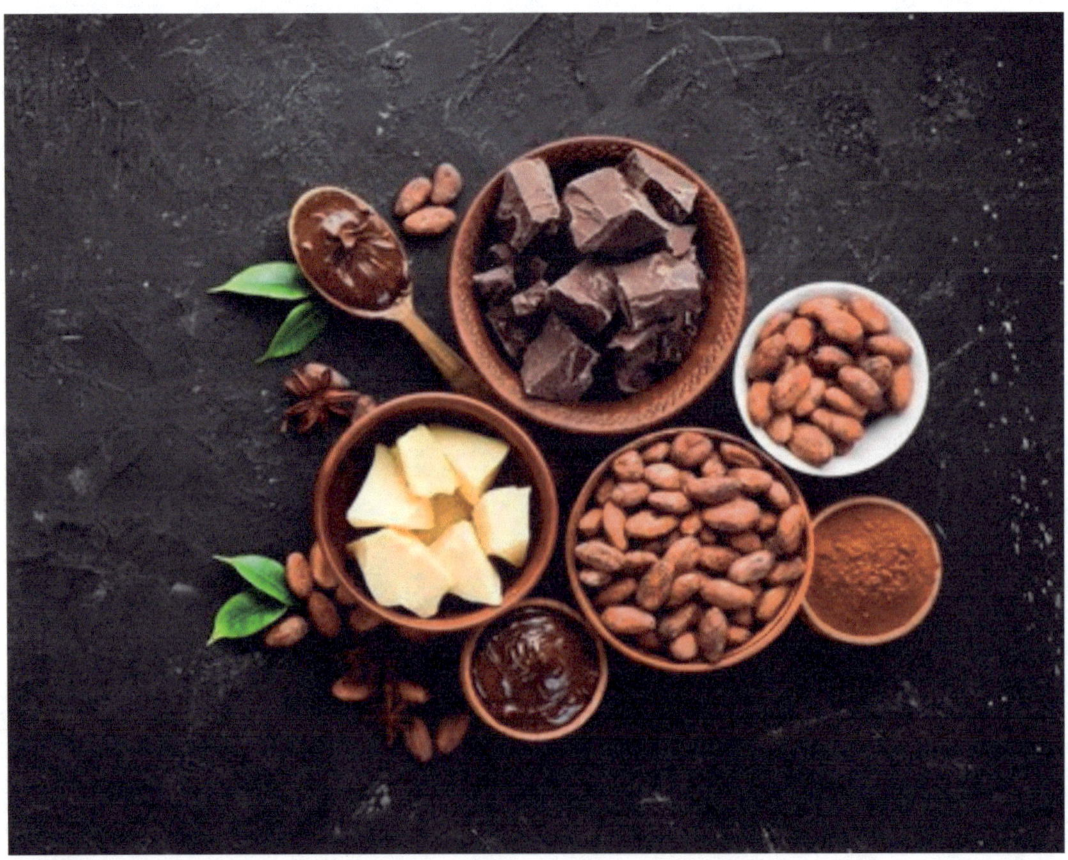

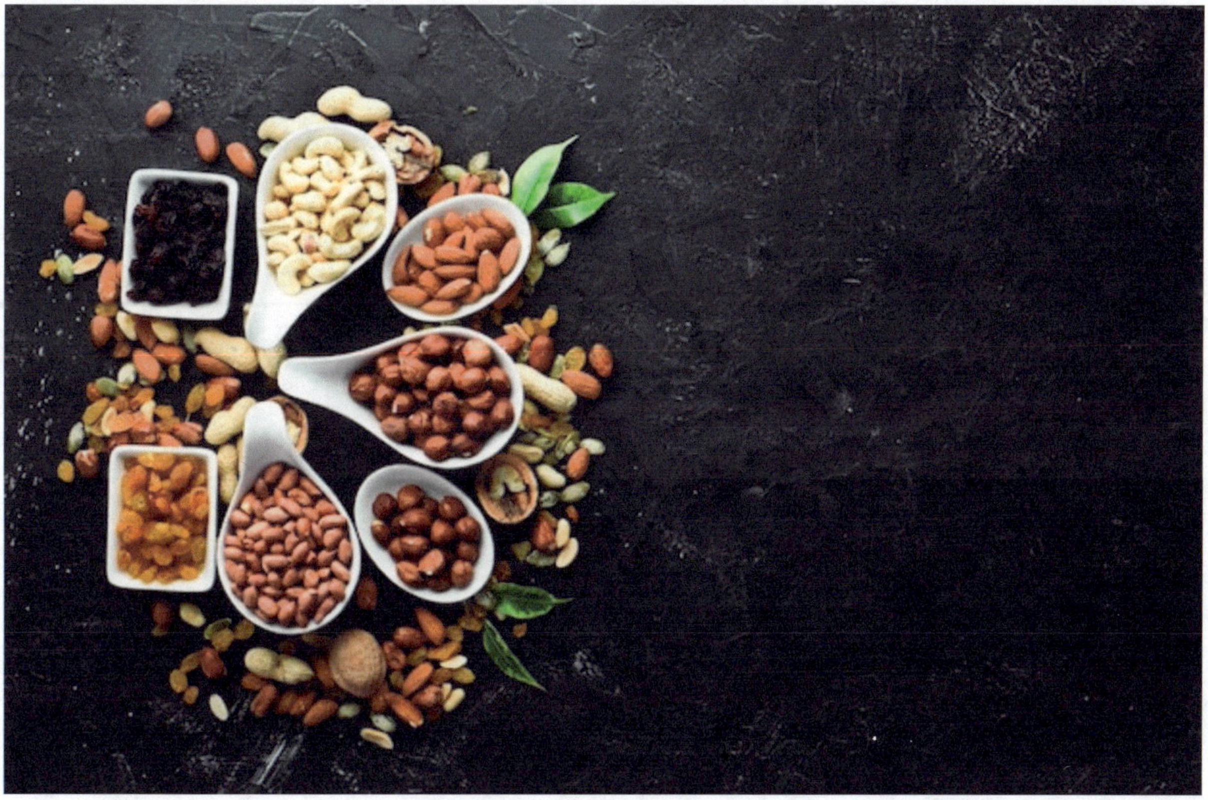

63. Spiced Nuts with Rosemary

Prep.Time:	Cook Time:	Serving:	Beverage pairing:
5 min	10-15 min	1	Black Coffee

Ingredients:

- 1 cup mixed nuts (such as almonds, cashews, walnuts)
- 1 tablespoon olive oil
- 1 tablespoon fresh rosemary, chopped
- 1/2 teaspoon ground cumin
- 1/4 teaspoon cayenne pepper
- Salt to taste

Preparation:

1. Preheat the oven to 350°F (175°C).
2. In a bowl, toss mixed nuts with olive oil, chopped rosemary, ground cumin, cayenne pepper, and salt until evenly coated.
3. Spread the spiced nuts on a baking sheet in a single layer.
4. Roast in the preheated oven for 10-15 minutes, stirring occasionally, until golden and fragrant.
5. Let cool before serving.

Nutrient Facts (per serving):

- Calories: Approximately 150 per serving
- Carbohydrates: 6g
- Fat: 12g
- Protein: 5g

64. Cinnamon Raisin Rice Cakes with Cream Cheese

Prep.Time:	Cook Time:	Serving:	Beverage pairing:
2 min	0 min	1	Tea

Ingredients:

- 2 rice cakes (sugar-free)
- 2 tablespoons cream cheese (low-fat or non-fat)
- 1/2 teaspoon ground cinnamon
- 2 tablespoons raisins

Preparation:

1. Spread cream cheese evenly on each rice cake.
2. Sprinkle ground cinnamon over the cream cheese.
3. Top with raisins.

Nutrient Facts (per serving):

- Calories: Approximately 120 per serving
- Carbohydrates: 18g
- Fat: 3g
- Protein: 2g

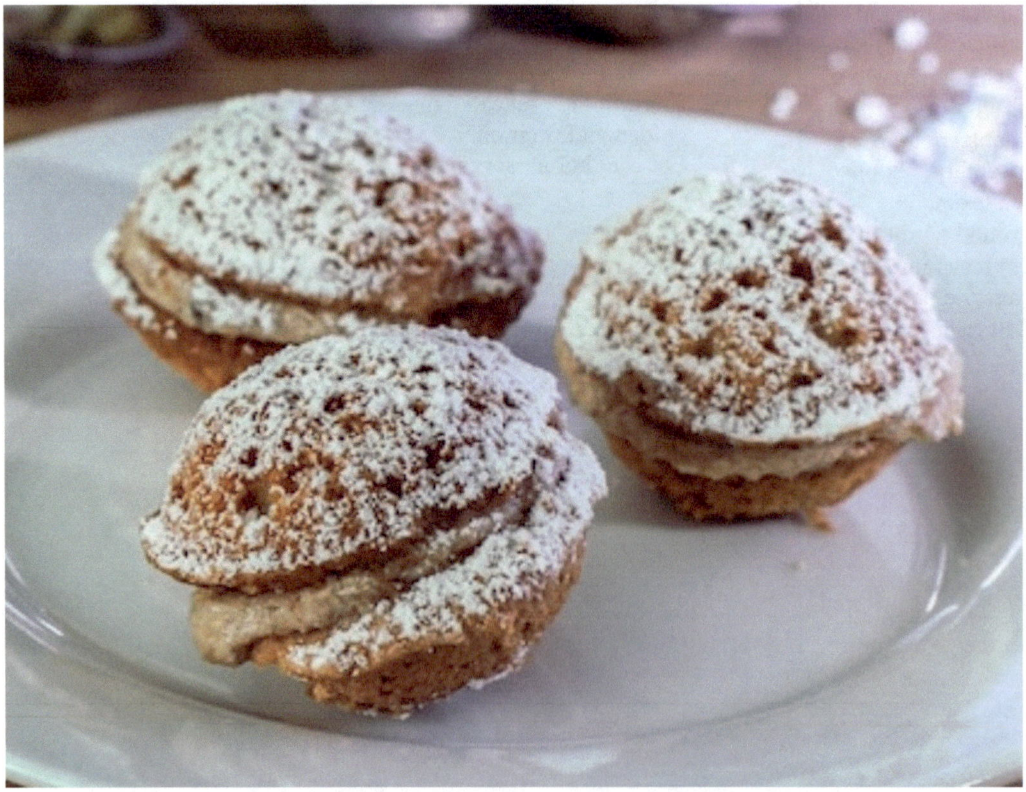

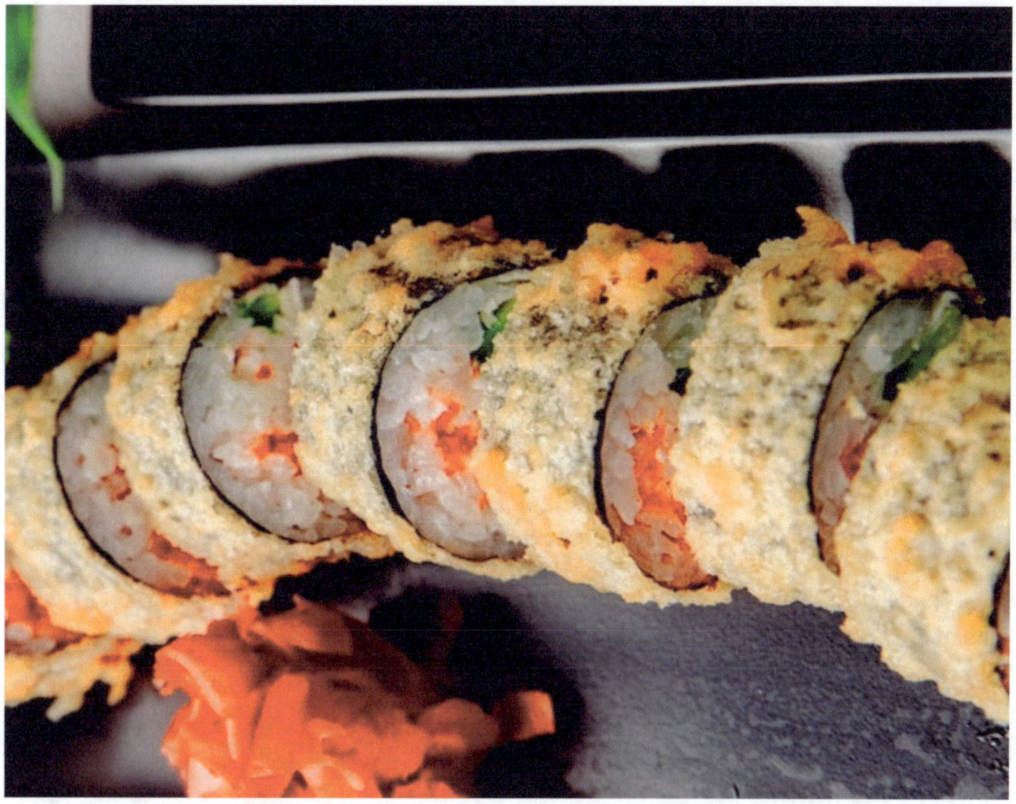

65. Vegetable Sushi Rolls with Brown Rice

Prep.Time: 15 min

Cook Time: 20 min

Serving: 1

Beverage pairing: Mint Water

Ingredients:

- 2 nori seaweed sheets
- 1 cup cooked brown rice
- Assorted vegetables (such as cucumber, avocado, carrot, bell pepper)

Soy sauce or tamari for dipping (low-sodium)

Preparation:

1. Place a nori seaweed sheet on a bamboo sushi mat or flat surface.
2. Spread cooked brown rice evenly over the nori sheet, leaving a small border along the edges.
3. Arrange thinly sliced vegetables in a row along the bottom edge of the rice.
4. Roll the nori sheet tightly around the filling, using the sushi mat to help shape the roll.
5. Slice the sushi roll into bite-sized pieces using a sharp knife.
6. Serve with soy sauce or tamari for dipping.

Nutrient Facts (per serving):

- Calories: Approximately 150 per serving
- Carbohydrates: 30g
- Fat: 2g
- Protein: 5g

66. Avocado and Tomato Salsa with Whole Grain Chips

Prep.Time:	Cook Time:	Serving:	Beverage pairing:
10 min	0 min	1	Cucumber Water

Ingredients:

- 1 ripe avocado, diced
- 1 tomato, diced
- 1/4 onion, finely chopped
- 1 tablespoon lime juice
- 1 tablespoon chopped cilantro
- Salt and pepper to taste
- Whole grain tortilla chips (sugar-free)

Preparation:

1. In a bowl, gently mix together diced avocado, diced tomato, finely chopped onion, lime juice, chopped cilantro, salt, and pepper.
2. Serve the avocado and tomato salsa with whole grain tortilla chips for dipping.

Nutrient Facts (per serving):

- Calories: Approximately 150 per serving
- Carbohydrates: 20g
- Fat: 8g
- Protein: 3g

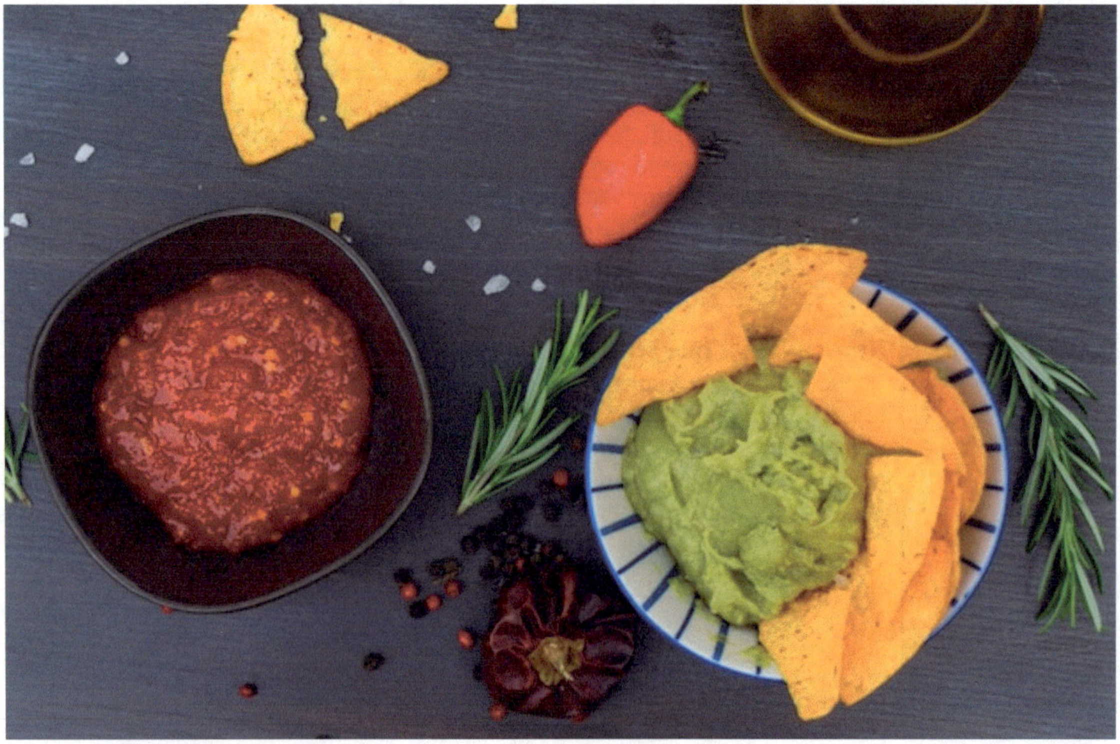

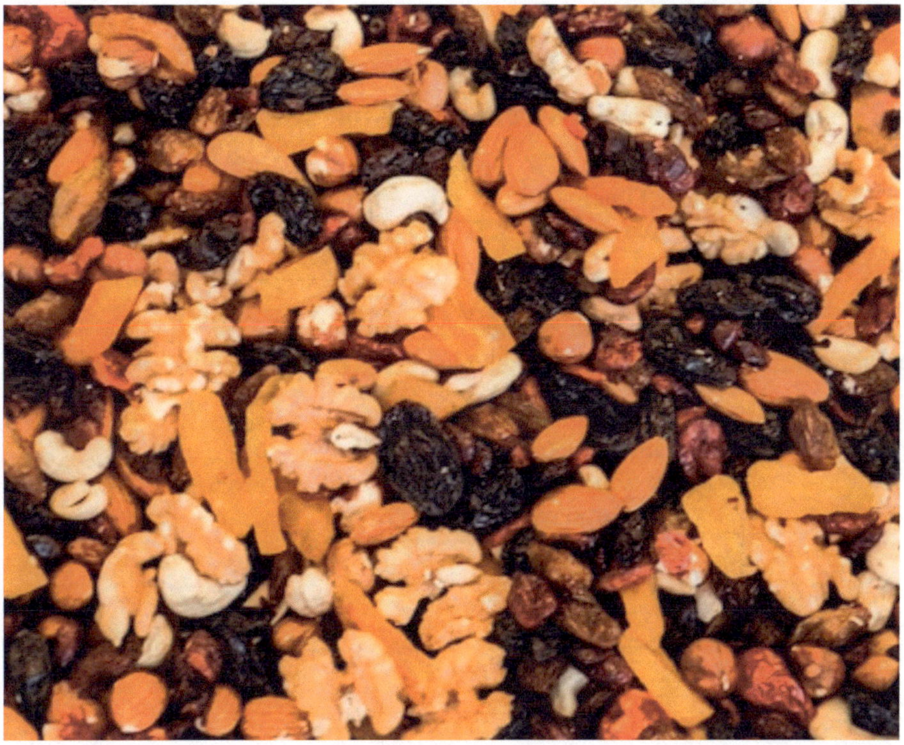

67. Pumpkin Seeds and Cranberry Snack Mix

Prep.Time: 2 min

Cook Time: 0 min

Serving: 1

Beverage pairing: Black Coffee

Ingredients:

- 1/4 cup pumpkin seeds
- 2 tablespoons dried cranberries (unsweetened)
- 1 tablespoon dark chocolate chips (sugar-free)

Preparation:

1. In a bowl, mix together pumpkin seeds, dried cranberries, and dark chocolate chips.
2. Enjoy as a nutritious snack.

Nutrient Facts (per serving):

- Calories: Approximately 120 per serving
- Carbohydrates: 10g
- Fat: 7g
- Protein: 5g

68. Sliced Pear with Almond Butter

Prep.Time:	Cook Time:	Serving:	Beverage pairing:
2 min	0 min	1	Black Tea

Ingredients:

- 1 ripe pear, sliced
- 2 tablespoons almond butter (unsweetened)

Preparation:

1. Arrange sliced pear on a plate.
2. Serve with almond butter for dipping or spreading.

Nutrient Facts (per serving):

- Calories: Approximately 150 per serving
- Carbohydrates: 20g
- Fat: 8g
- Protein: 3g

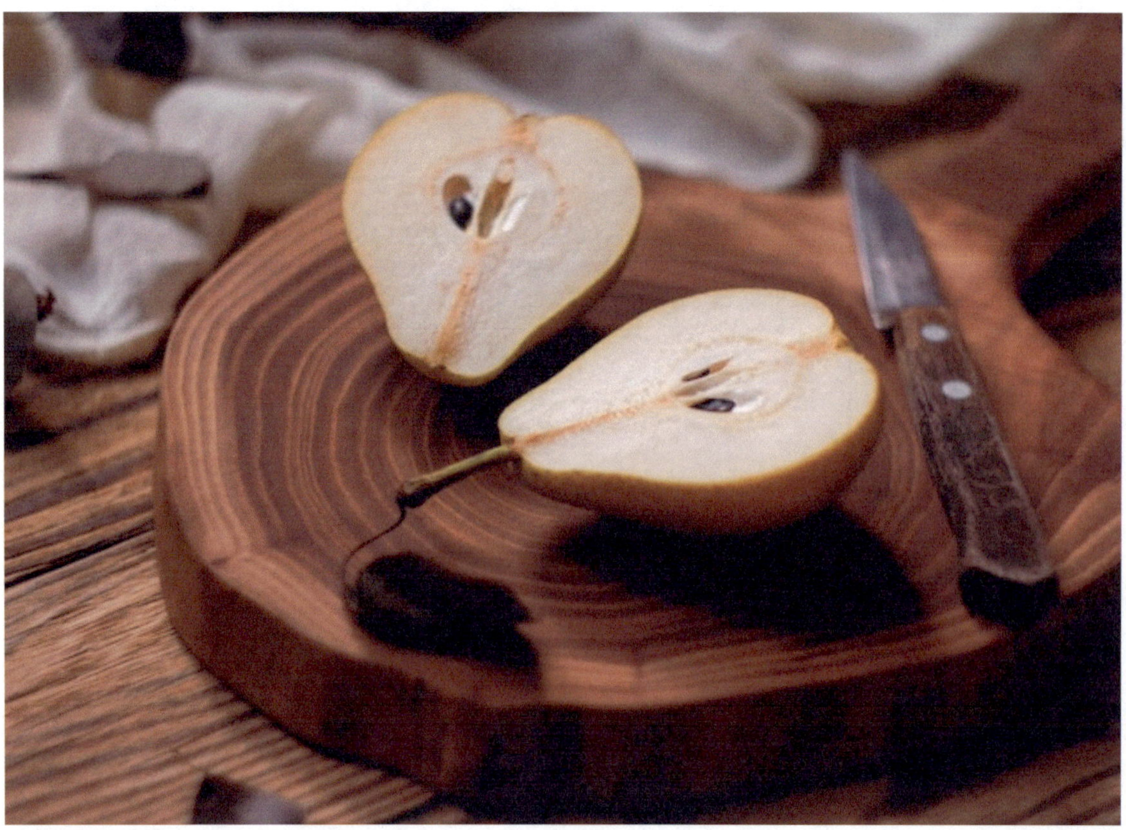

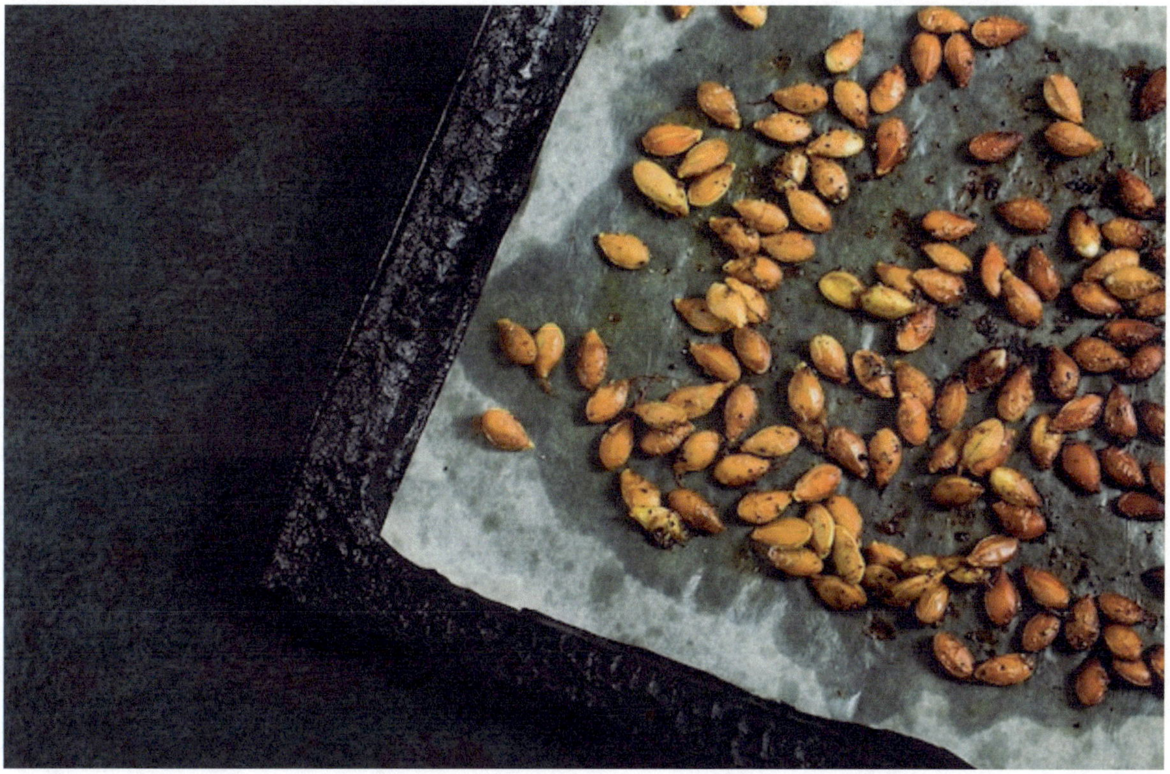

69. Cajun Roasted Pumpkin Seeds

Prep.Time: 5 min

Cook Time: 20-25 min

Serving: 1

Beverage pairing: Mint Water

Ingredients:

- 1 cup raw pumpkin seeds (pepitas)
- 1 tablespoon olive oil
- 1 teaspoon Cajun seasoning
- 1/2 teaspoon garlic powder
- 1/4 teaspoon salt

Preparation:

1. Preheat the oven to 300°F (150°C). Line a baking sheet with parchment paper.
2. In a bowl, toss together raw pumpkin seeds, olive oil, Cajun seasoning, garlic powder, and salt until the seeds are well coated.
3. Spread the seasoned pumpkin seeds in an even layer on the prepared baking sheet.
4. Roast in the preheated oven for 20-25 minutes, stirring occasionally, until the seeds are golden brown and crispy.
5. Remove from the oven and let cool completely before serving or storing in an airtight container.
6. Enjoy these flavorful Cajun Roasted Pumpkin Seeds as a crunchy and nutritious snack.

Nutrient Facts (per serving):

- Calories: Approximately 120 per serving (1/4 cup)
- Carbohydrates: 3g
- Fat: 10g
- Protein: 5g

70. Roasted Garlic and Herb Chickpea Snack

Prep.Time:	Cook Time:	Serving:	Beverage pairing:
5 min	20-25 min	1	Water

Ingredients:

- 1 can (15 ounces) chickpeas, drained and rinsed
- 1 tablespoon olive oil
- 1 teaspoon garlic powder
- 1 teaspoon dried mixed herbs (such as rosemary, thyme, oregano)
- Salt and pepper to taste

Preparation:

1. Preheat the oven to 400°F (200°C).
2. Pat the chickpeas dry with paper towels and spread them on a baking sheet.
3. Drizzle olive oil over the chickpeas and sprinkle with garlic powder, dried mixed herbs, salt, and pepper. Toss until evenly coated.
4. Roast in the preheated oven for 20-25 minutes, shaking the pan halfway through, until crispy.
5. Let cool before serving.

Nutrient Facts (per serving):

- Calories: Approximately 150 per serving
- Carbohydrates: 20g
- Fat: 5g
- Protein: 7g

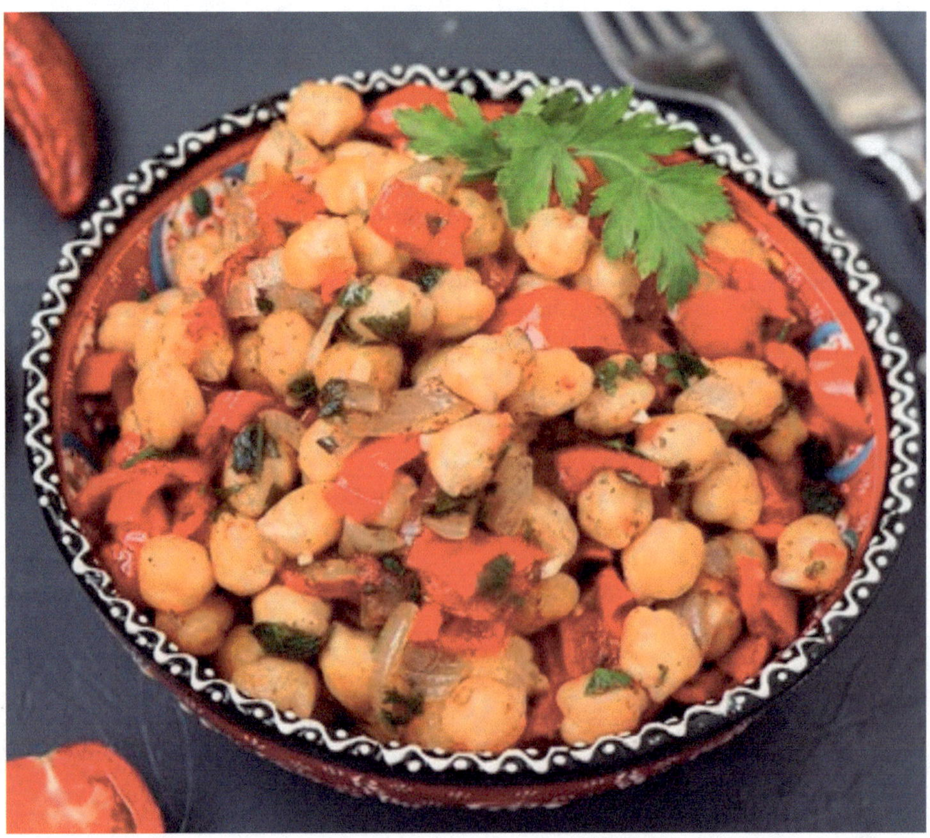

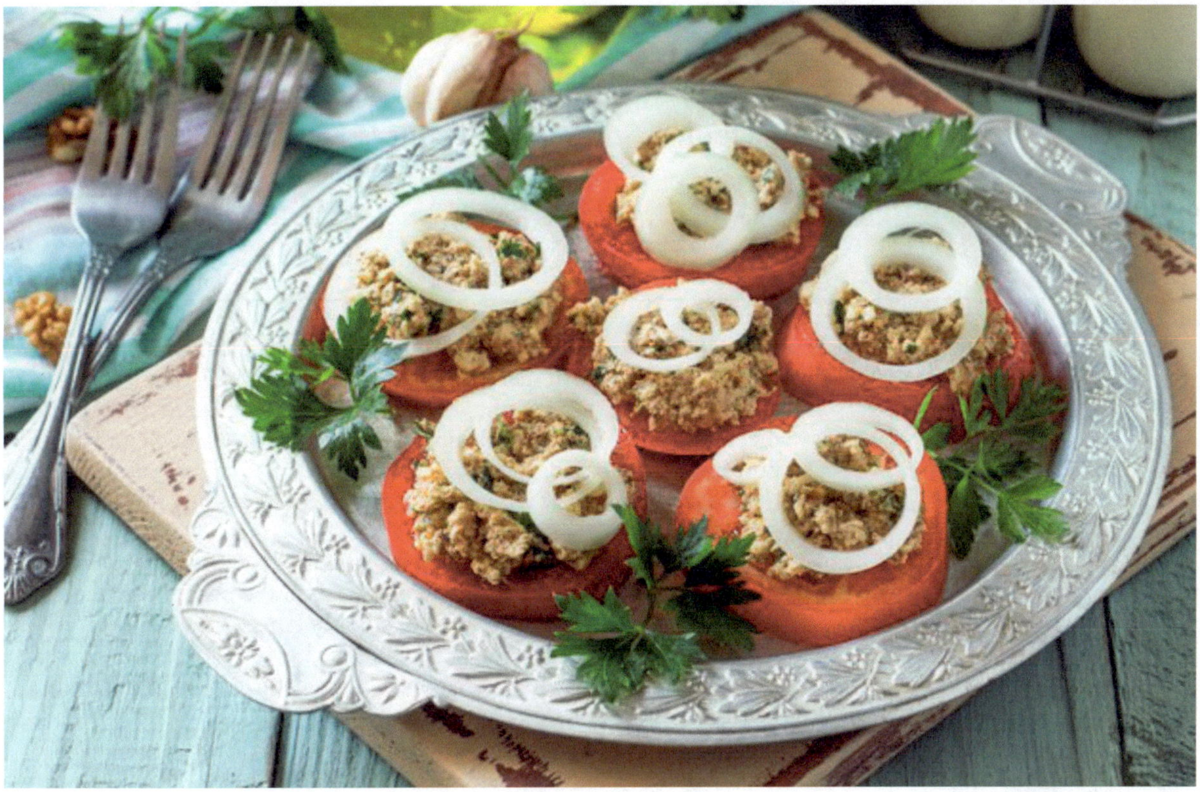

71. Stuffed Cherry Tomatoes with Tuna Salad

Prep.Time: 10 min

Cook Time: 0 min

Serving: 1

Beverage pairing: Black Tea

Ingredients:

- Cherry tomatoes
- 1 can (5 ounces) tuna, drained
- 2 tablespoons mayonnaise (preferably sugar-free)
- 1 tablespoon diced red onion
- 1 tablespoon diced celery
- Salt and pepper to taste

Preparation:

1. Slice the tops off cherry tomatoes and scoop out the seeds.
2. In a bowl, mix together drained tuna, mayonnaise, diced red onion, diced celery, salt, and pepper.
3. Spoon the tuna salad into the hollowed-out cherry tomatoes.
4. Serve as appetizers or snacks.

Nutrient Facts (per serving):

- Calories: Approximately 100 per serving
- Carbohydrates: 3g
- Fat: 5g
- Protein: 10g

72. Quinoa-Stuffed Bell Peppers

Prep.Time:	Cook Time:	Serving:	Beverage pairing:
20 min	25-30 min	1	Green Water

Ingredients:

- 4 large bell peppers (any color)
- 1 cup cooked quinoa
- 1 can (15 ounces) black beans, drained and rinsed
- 1 cup corn kernels (fresh, frozen, or canned)
- 1/2 cup diced tomatoes
- 1 teaspoon ground cumin
- 1 teaspoon chili powder
- Salt and pepper to taste
- Fresh cilantro leaves for garnish (optional)

Preparation:

1. Preheat the oven to 375°F (190°C). Cut the tops off the bell peppers and remove the seeds and membranes.
2. In a large bowl, mix together cooked quinoa, black beans, corn kernels, diced tomatoes, shredded cheddar cheese if using, ground cumin, chili powder, salt, and pepper.
3. Stuff each bell pepper with the quinoa mixture, pressing down gently to pack it in.
4. Place the stuffed bell peppers in a baking dish. Cover with foil and bake in the preheated oven for 25-30 minutes, or until the peppers are tender.
5. Remove from the oven and let cool slightly before serving.
6. Garnish with fresh cilantro leaves if desired.
7. Enjoy these flavorful and nutritious Quinoa-Stuffed Bell Peppers as a satisfying meal or snack.

Nutrient Facts (per serving):

- Calories: Approximately 200 per serving (1 stuffed pepper)
- Carbohydrates: 30g
- Fat: 5g
- Protein: 10g

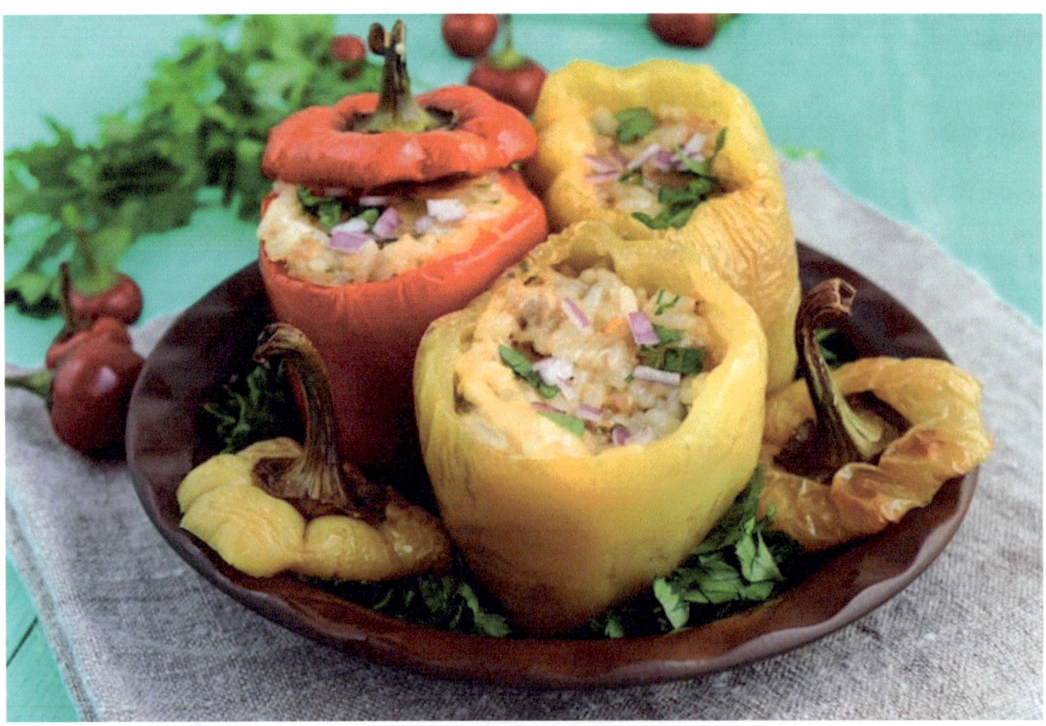

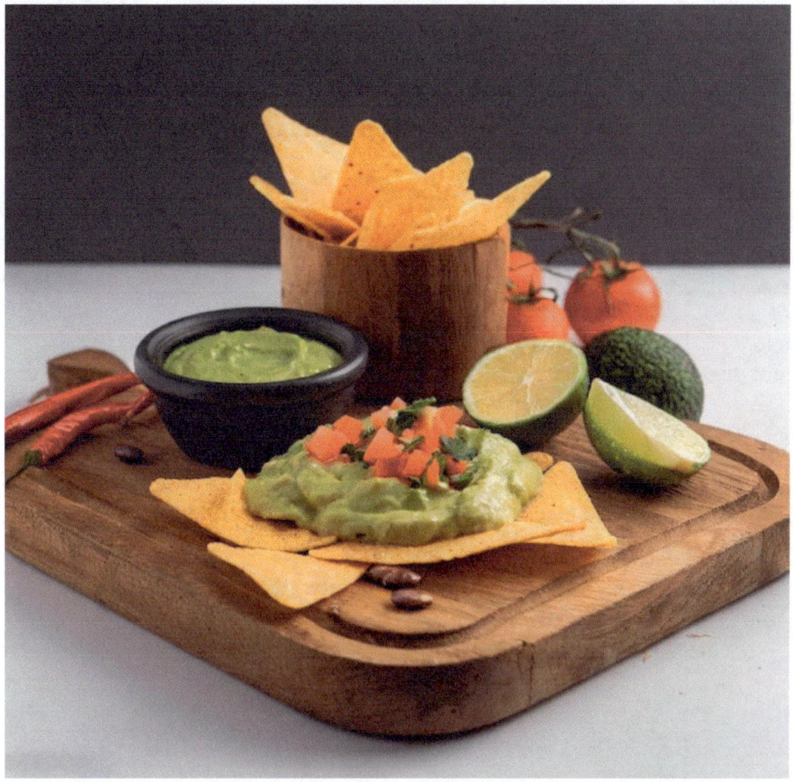

73. Bell Pepper Nachos with Guacamole

Prep.Time: 10 min

Cook Time: 10-12 min

Serving: 1

Beverage pairing: Lemonade

Ingredients:

- Bell peppers, sliced into rings
- 1/2 cup shredded cheese (such as cheddar or mozzarella)
- 1/4 cup diced tomatoes
- 1/4 cup diced onions
- Guacamole for topping

Preparation:

1. Preheat the oven to 375°F (190°C).
2. Arrange bell pepper rings on a baking sheet lined with parchment paper.
3. Sprinkle shredded cheese evenly over the bell pepper rings.
4. Top with diced tomatoes and onions.
5. Bake in the preheated oven for 10-12 minutes, or until the cheese is melted and bubbly.
6. Serve with guacamole for dipping.

Nutrient Facts (per serving):

- Calories: Approximately 150 per serving
- Carbohydrates: 10g
- Fat: 10g
- Protein: 5g

74. Cottage Cheese and Sliced Strawberries

Prep.Time: 10 min

Cook Time: 0 min

Serving: 1

Beverage pairing: Herbal Tea

Ingredients:

- 1/2 cup cottage cheese (low-fat or non-fat)
- Sliced strawberries

Preparation:

1. Spoon cottage cheese into a bowl.
2. Top with sliced strawberries.
3. Serve as a simple and nutritious snack.

Nutrient Facts (per serving):

- Calories: Approximately 100 per serving
- Carbohydrates: 10g
- Fat: 2g
  Protein: 10g

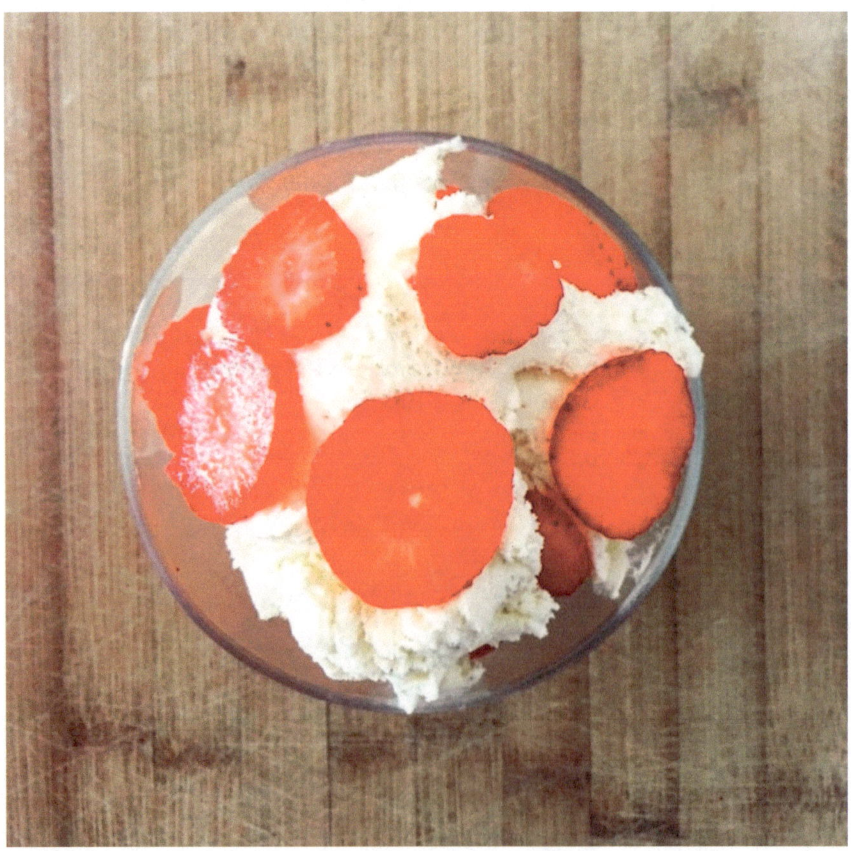

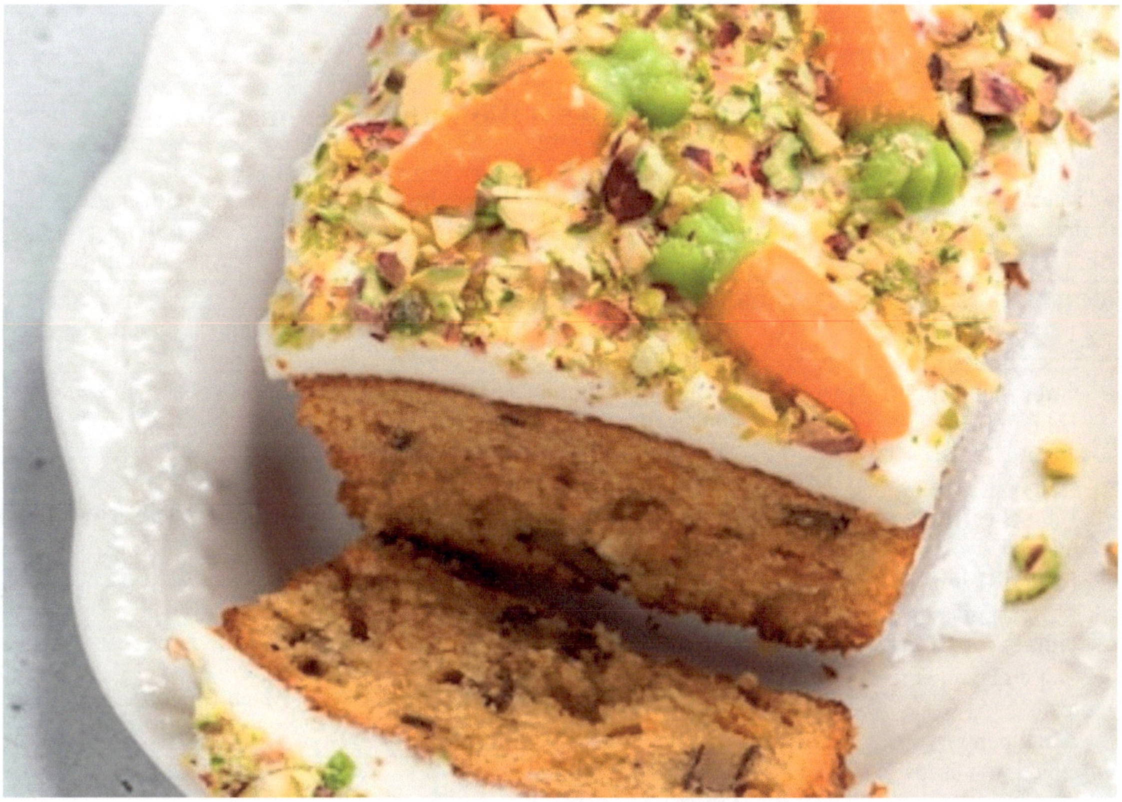

75. Apricot and Pistachio Rice Cakes

Prep.Time: 5 min

Cook Time: 0 min

Serving: 1

Beverage pairing: Coconut Water

Ingredients:

- 4 rice cakes
- 1/4 cup unsweetened almond butter or peanut butter
- 1/4 cup dried apricots, chopped
- 2 tablespoons pistachios, chopped
- Honey or maple syrup for drizzling (optional)

Preparation:

1. Spread almond butter or peanut butter evenly over each rice cake.
2. Sprinkle chopped dried apricots and pistachios over the almond butter or peanut butter layer.
3. If desired, drizzle honey or maple syrup over the toppings for added sweetness.
4. Serve immediately and enjoy these Apricot and Pistachio Rice Cakes as a delicious and satisfying snack.

Nutrient Facts (per serving):

- Calories: Approximately 150 per serving (2 rice cakes)
- Carbohydrates: 20g
- Fat: 6g
- Protein: 3g

76. Cilantro Lime Black Bean Dip with Bell Pepper Strips

Prep.Time:	Cook Time:	Serving:	Beverage pairing:
10 min	0 min	1	Lemonade

Ingredients:

- 1 can (15 ounces) black beans, drained and rinsed
- 1/4 cup fresh cilantro leaves, chopped
- 1 clove garlic, minced
- Juice of 1 lime
- 1/2 teaspoon ground cumin
- Salt and pepper to taste
- 2 bell peppers, sliced into strips for dipping

Preparation:

1. In a food processor, combine black beans, chopped cilantro leaves, minced garlic, lime juice, ground cumin, salt, and pepper.
2. Blend until smooth, scraping down the sides as needed, to achieve desired consistency.
3. Transfer the black bean dip to a serving bowl.
4. Serve with sliced bell peppers for dipping.
5. Enjoy this flavorful and nutritious Cilantro Lime Black Bean Dip with Bell Pepper Strips as a healthy snack or appetizer.

Nutrient Facts (per serving):

- Calories: Approximately 100 per serving (2 tablespoons dip with bell pepper strips)
- Carbohydrates: 12g
- Fat: 4g
- Protein: 4g

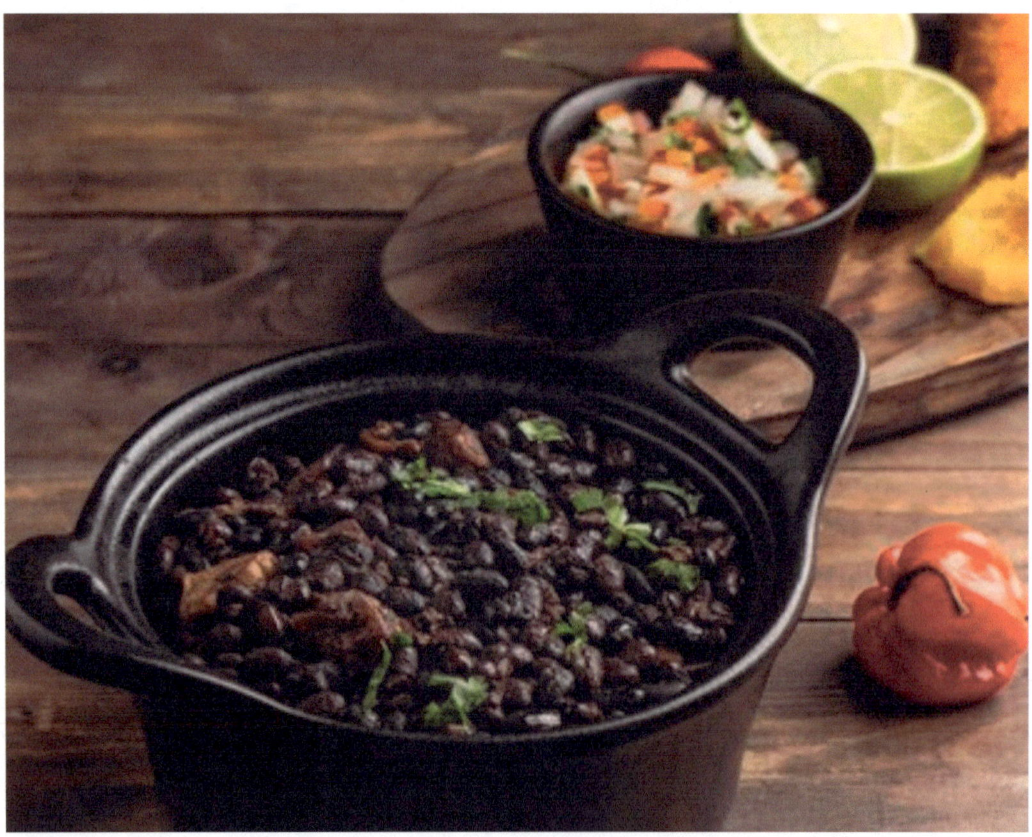

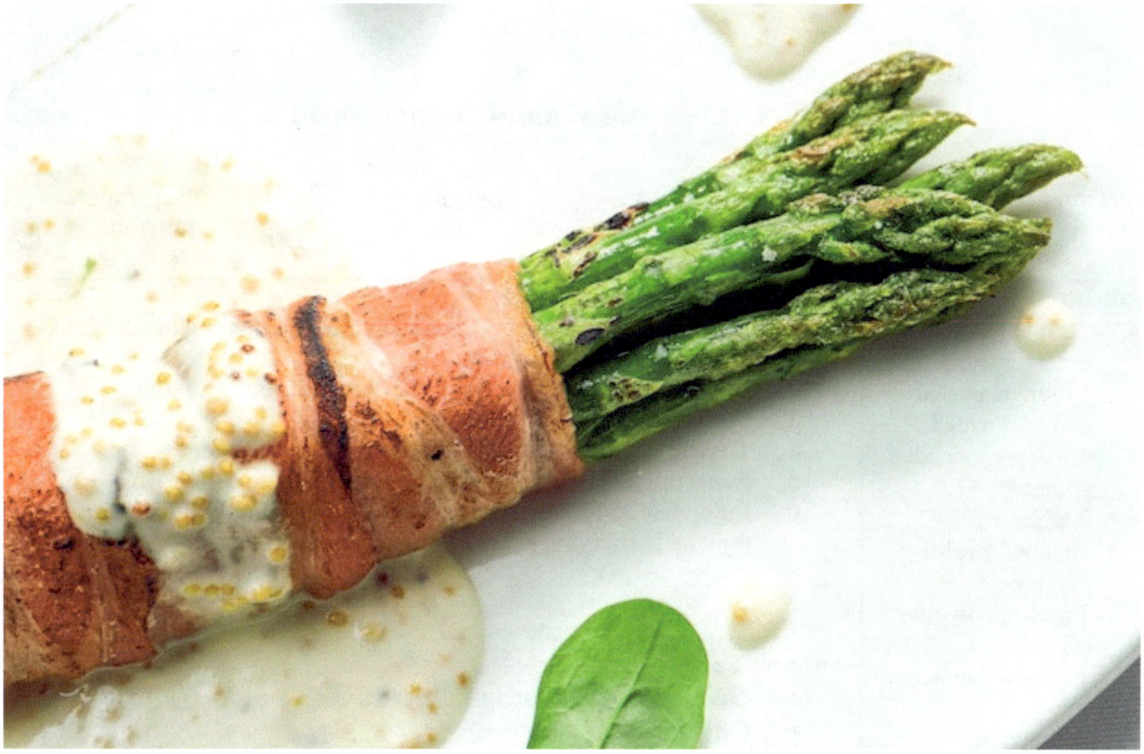

77. Roasted Asparagus Spears with Parmesan

Prep.Time: 5 min | **Cook Time:** 10-12 min | **Serving:** 1 | **Beverage pairing:** Black Coffee

Ingredients:

- Fresh asparagus spears
- 1 tablespoon olive oil
- Salt and pepper to taste
- Grated Parmesan cheese

Preparation:

1. Preheat the oven to 400°F (200°C).
2. Trim the tough ends off the asparagus spears.
3. Arrange the asparagus spears on a baking sheet lined with parchment paper.
4. Drizzle olive oil over the asparagus and season with salt and pepper.
5. Roast in the preheated oven for 10-12 minutes, or until tender.
6. Sprinkle grated Parmesan cheese over the roasted asparagus before serving.

Nutrient Facts (per serving):

- Calories: Approximately 100 per serving
- Carbohydrates: 6g
- Fat: 7g
- Protein: 5g

78. Orange and Walnut Quinoa Salad

Prep.Time: 15 min

Cook Time: 0 min

Serving: 1

Beverage pairing: Iced Tea

Ingredients:

- 1 cup cooked quinoa
- 1 orange, peeled and segmented
- 1/4 cup chopped walnuts
- 2 tablespoons chopped fresh parsley
- 1 tablespoon olive oil
- 1 tablespoon lemon juice
- Salt and pepper to taste

Preparation:

1. In a large bowl, combine cooked quinoa, orange segments, chopped walnuts, and chopped fresh parsley.
2. Drizzle olive oil and lemon juice over the quinoa mixture.
3. Season with salt and pepper to taste.
4. Toss gently until all ingredients are well combined.
5. Serve immediately or refrigerate until ready to serve.
6. Enjoy this refreshing and nutritious Orange and Walnut Quinoa Salad as a light and satisfying snack or side dish.

Nutrient Facts (per serving):

- Calories: Approximately 180 per serving (1 cup)
- Carbohydrates: 22g
- Fat: 8g
- Protein: 5g

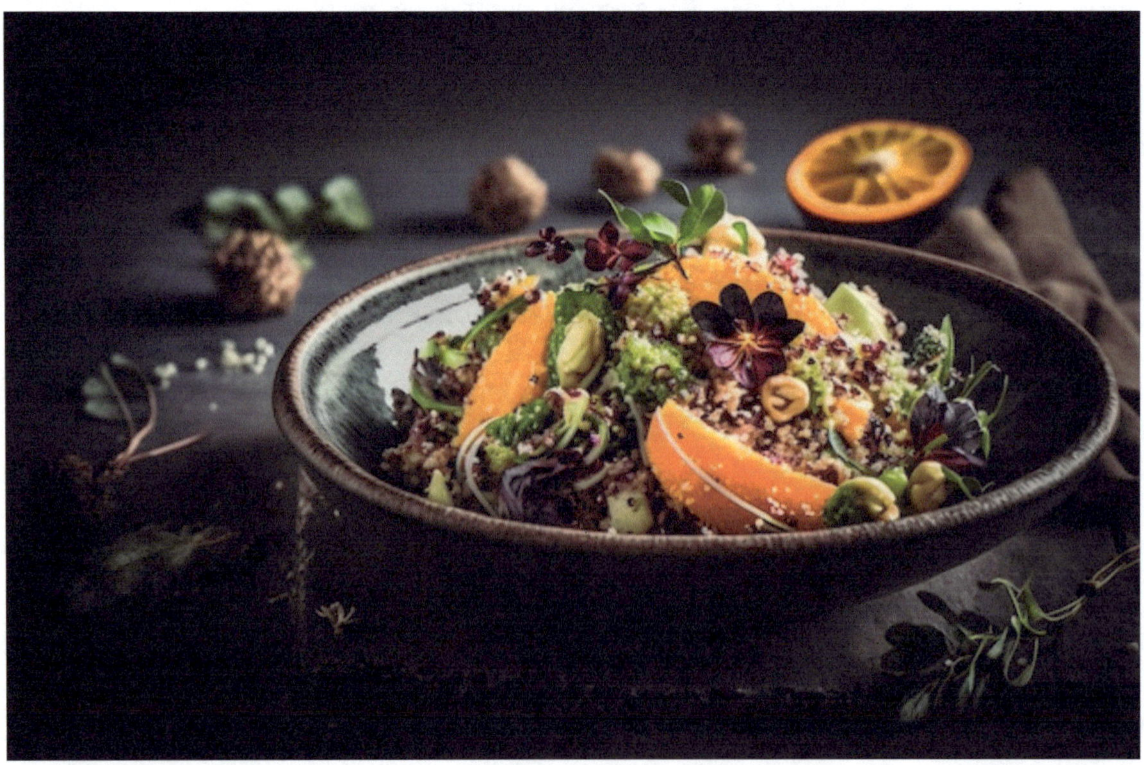

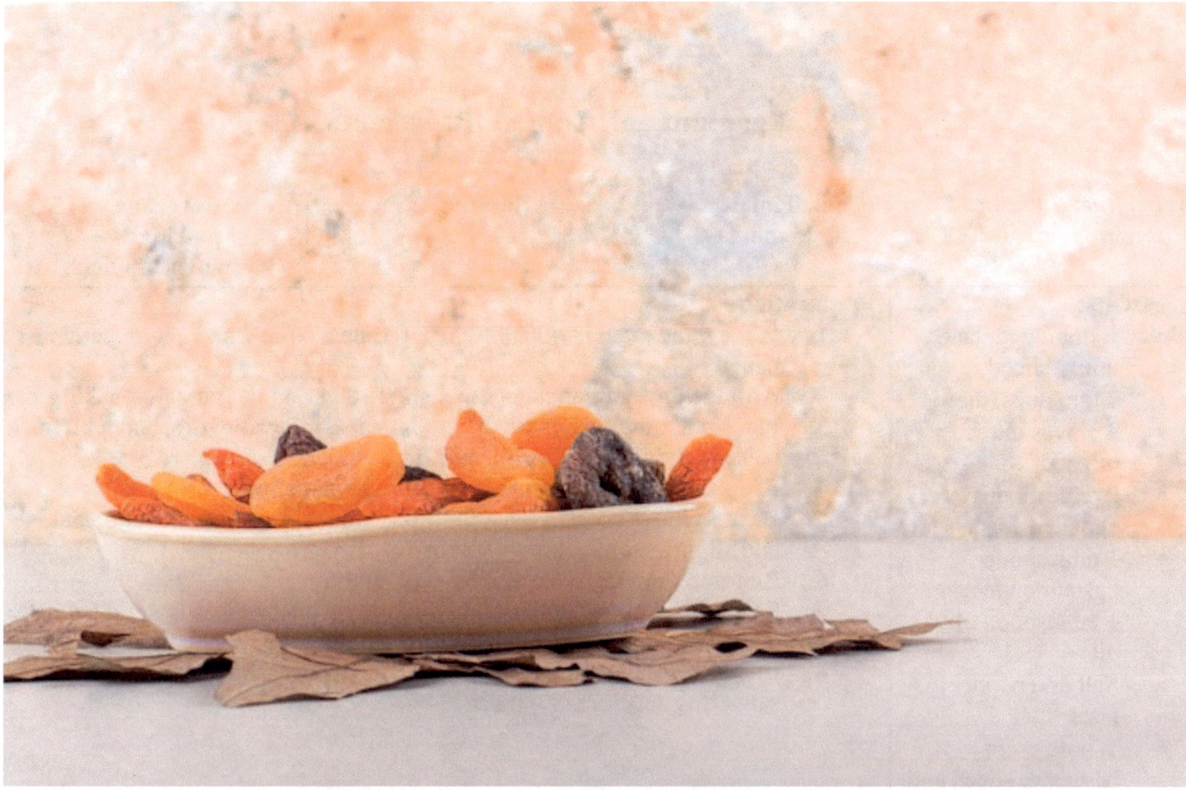

79. Pistachios and Dried Apricots Combo

Prep.Time: 2 min | **Cook Time:** 0 min | **Serving:** 1 | **Beverage pairing:** Black Coffee

Ingredients:

- 1/4 cup pistachios
- 1/4 cup dried apricots (unsweetened)

Preparation:

1. Combine pistachios and dried apricots in a bowl.
2. Enjoy as a satisfying and nutritious snack.

Nutrient Facts (per serving):

- Calories: Approximately 150 per serving
- Carbohydrates: 15g
- Fat: 9g
- Protein: 4g

80. Eggplant and Tomato Bruschetta

Prep.Time: 15 min

Cook Time: 20-25 min

Serving: 1

Beverage pairing: Veges. Juice

Ingredients:

- 1 small eggplant, thinly sliced
- 2 tomatoes, diced
- 2 cloves garlic, minced
- 2 tablespoons chopped fresh basil
- 1 tablespoon balsamic vinegar
- 1 tablespoon olive oil
- Salt and pepper to taste
- Whole grain baguette, sliced and toasted (optional)

Preparation:

1. Preheat the oven to 400°F (200°C). Line a baking sheet with parchment paper.
2. Arrange the eggplant slices in a single layer on the prepared baking sheet.
3. In a small bowl, combine diced tomatoes, minced garlic, chopped fresh basil, balsamic vinegar, olive oil, salt, and pepper.
4. Spoon the tomato mixture over the eggplant slices.
5. Bake in the preheated oven for 20-25 minutes, or until the eggplant is tender and slightly golden brown.
6. Remove from the oven and let cool slightly.
7. Serve the eggplant and tomato mixture on toasted whole grain baguette slices, if desired.
8. Enjoy this flavorful Eggplant and Tomato Bruschetta as a delicious and satisfying snack or appetizer.

Nutrient Facts (per serving):

- Calories: Approximately 120 per serving (2 slices)
- Carbohydrates: 15g
- Fat: 5g
- Protein: 3g

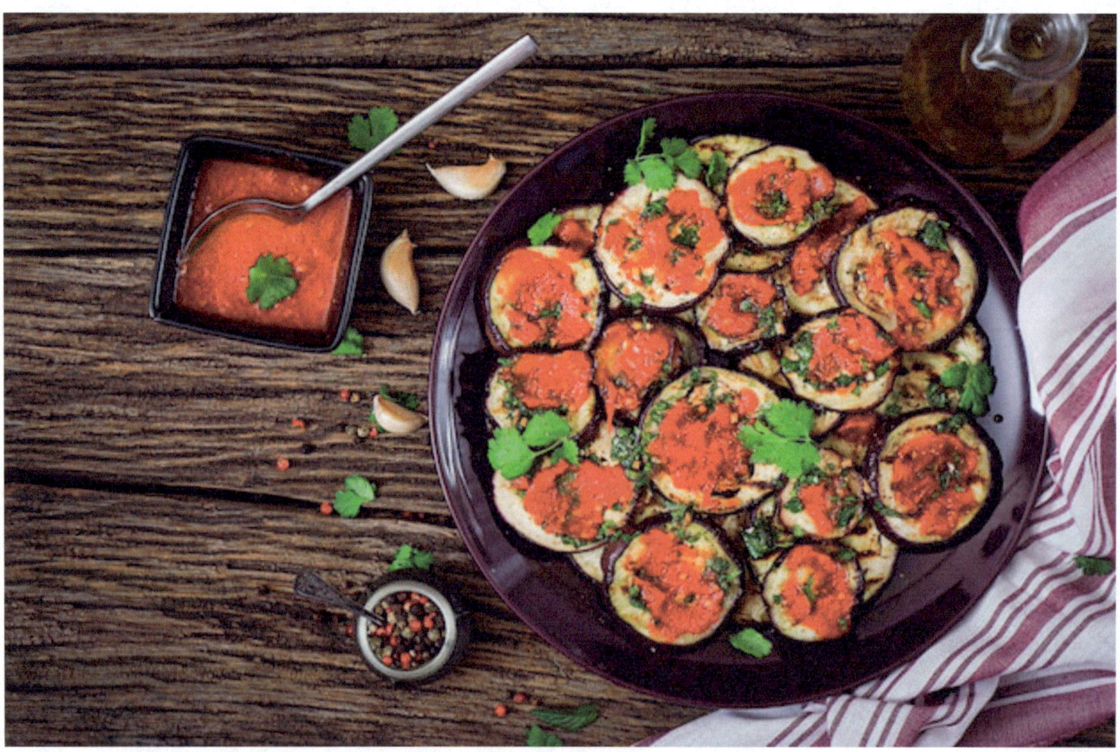

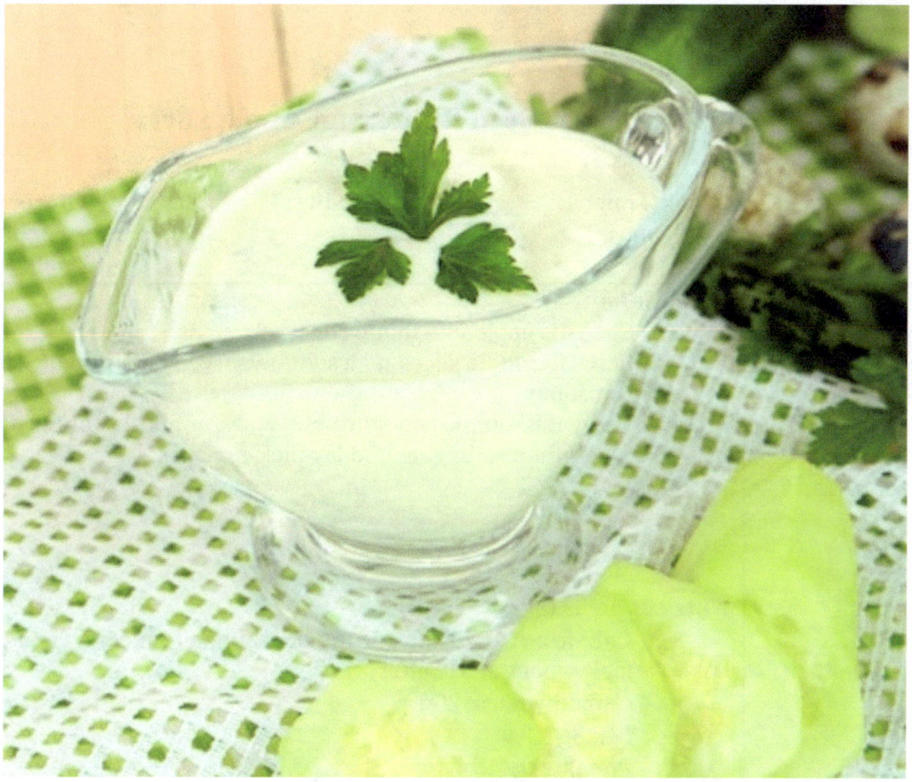

81. Minty Yogurt Cucumber Slices

Prep.Time: 5 min

Cook Time: 0 min

Serving: 1

Beverage pairing: Almond Milk

Ingredients:

- 1/2 cup plain Greek yogurt
- 2 tablespoons chopped fresh mint leaves
- 1 teaspoon lemon juice
- Salt and pepper to taste
- 1 cucumber, sliced

Preparation:

1. In a small bowl, mix together plain Greek yogurt, chopped fresh mint leaves, lemon juice, salt, and pepper until well combined.
2. Arrange cucumber slices on a serving plate.
3. Serve the minty yogurt dip alongside the cucumber slices.
4. Enjoy this refreshing and nutritious Minty Yogurt Cucumber Slices as a light and healthy snack.

Nutrient Facts (per serving):

- Calories: Approximately 50 per serving (4 slices with dip)
- Carbohydrates: 4g
- Fat: 2g
- Protein: 3g

82. Sunflower Seed Butter and Apple Slices

Prep.Time:	Cook Time:	Serving:	Beverage pairing:
5 min	0 min	1	Ginger Water

Ingredients:

- 1 medium apple, sliced
- 2 tablespoons sunflower seed butter

Preparation:

1. Slice the apple into thin wedges or rounds.
2. Serve the apple slices with sunflower seed butter on the side for dipping or spreading.
3. Enjoy this simple and nutritious snack of Sunflower Seed Butter and Apple Slices for a satisfying midday pick-me-up.

Nutrient Facts (per serving):

- Calories: Approximately 150 per serving (1 medium apple with 2 tablespoons seed butter)
- Carbohydrates: 20g
- Fat: 8g
- Protein: 3g

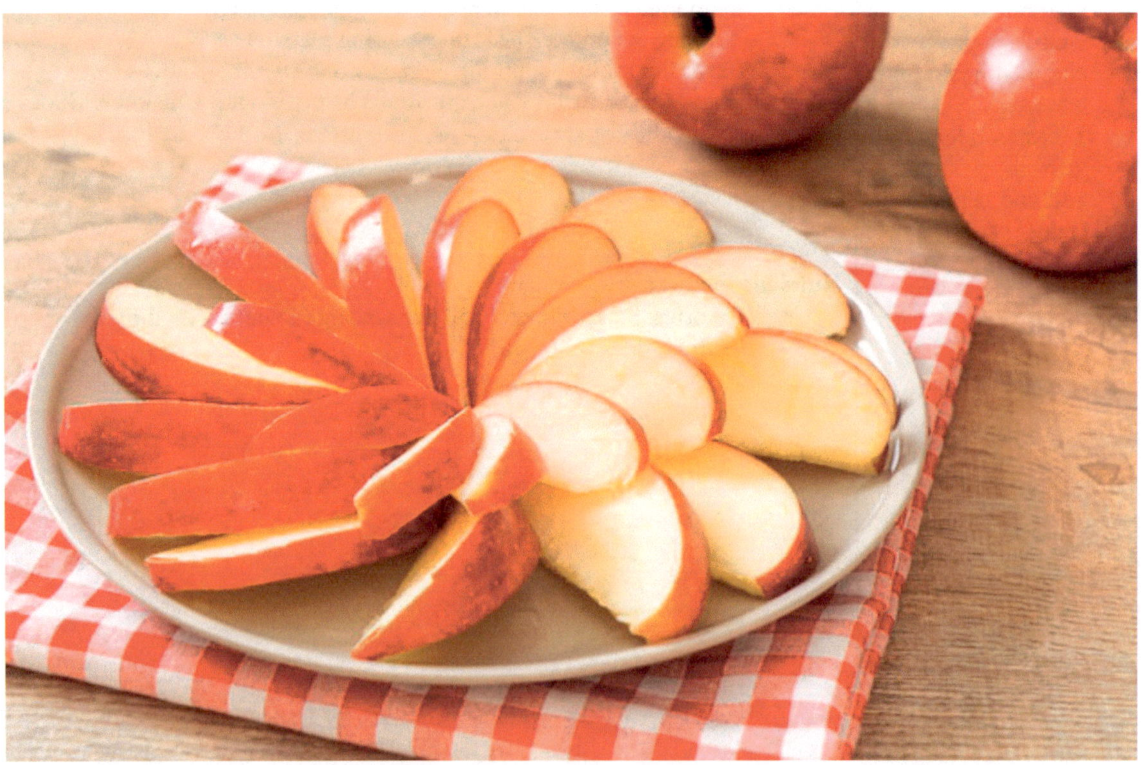

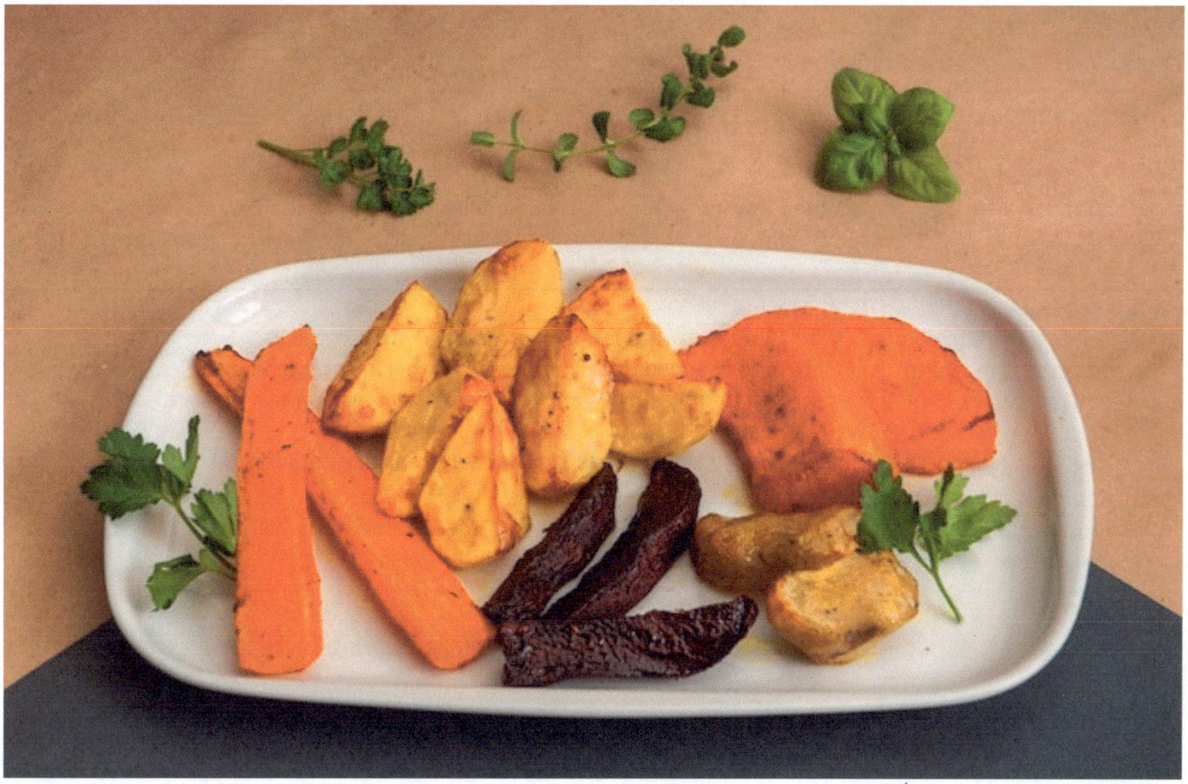

83. Homemade Vegetable Chips

Prep.Time:	Cook Time:	Serving:	Beverage pairing:
10 min	20-25 min	1	Mint Tea

Ingredients:

- 1 zucchini, thinly sliced
- 1 sweet potato, thinly sliced
- 1 beet, thinly sliced
- 1 tablespoon olive oil
- Salt and pepper to taste

Preparation:

1. Preheat the oven to 375°F (190°C).
2. In a bowl, toss thinly sliced zucchini, sweet potato, and beet with olive oil until evenly coated.
3. Arrange the vegetable slices in a single layer on baking sheets lined with parchment paper.
4. Sprinkle with salt and pepper to taste.
5. Bake in the preheated oven for 20-25 minutes, flipping halfway through, until crispy.
6. Let cool before serving

Nutrient Facts (per serving):

- Calories: Approximately 100 per serving
- Carbohydrates: 15g
- Fat: 4g
- Protein: 2g

84. Turkey and Avocado Lettuce Cups

Prep.Time: 5 min

Cook Time: 0 min

Serving: 1

Beverage pairing: Chamomile Tea

Ingredients:

- Large lettuce leaves (such as romaine or butter lettuce)
- Sliced turkey breast
- Sliced avocado
- Optional: Mustard or mayonnaise (sugar-free)

Preparation:

1. Lay out large lettuce leaves on a clean surface.
2. Place sliced turkey breast and sliced avocado on each lettuce leaf.
3. Optional: Spread mustard or mayonnaise on the turkey slices.
4. Roll up the lettuce leaves to form cups.
5. Serve as a light and protein-rich snack or appetizer.

Nutrient Facts (per serving):

- Calories: Approximately 150 per serving
- Carbohydrates: 5g
- Fat: 8g
- Protein: 15g

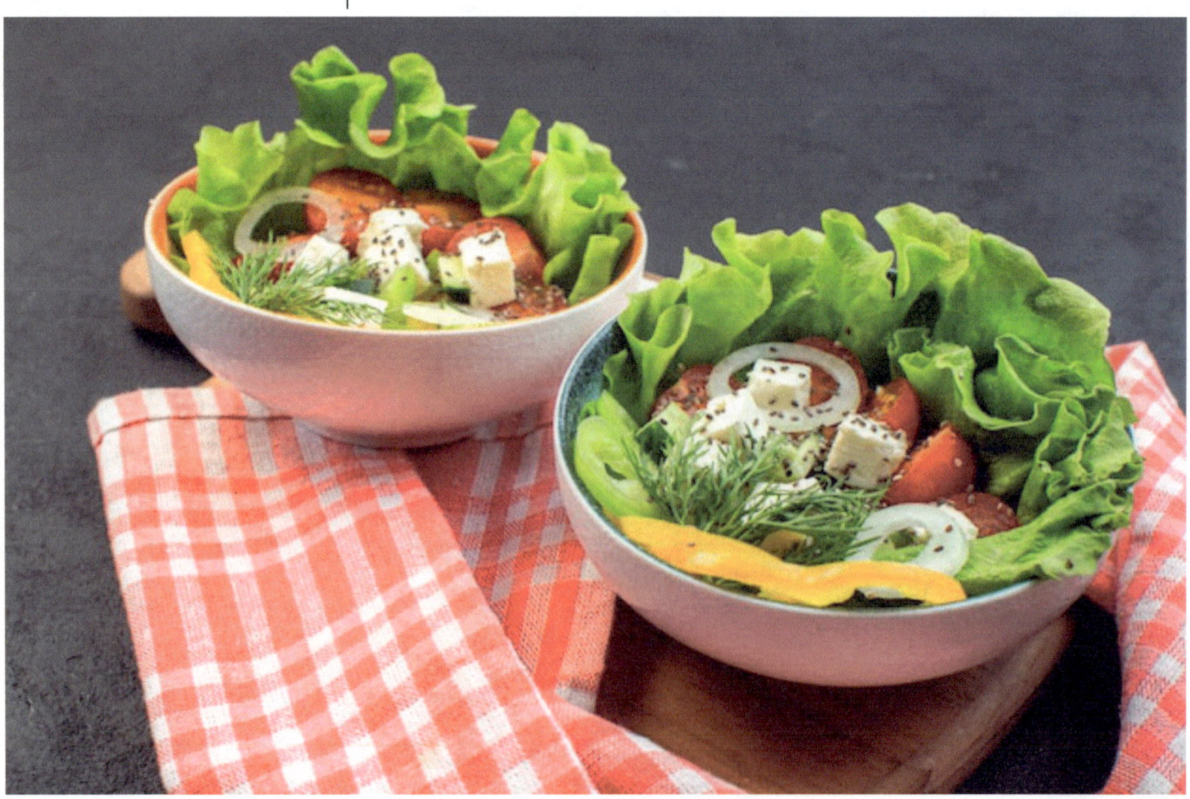

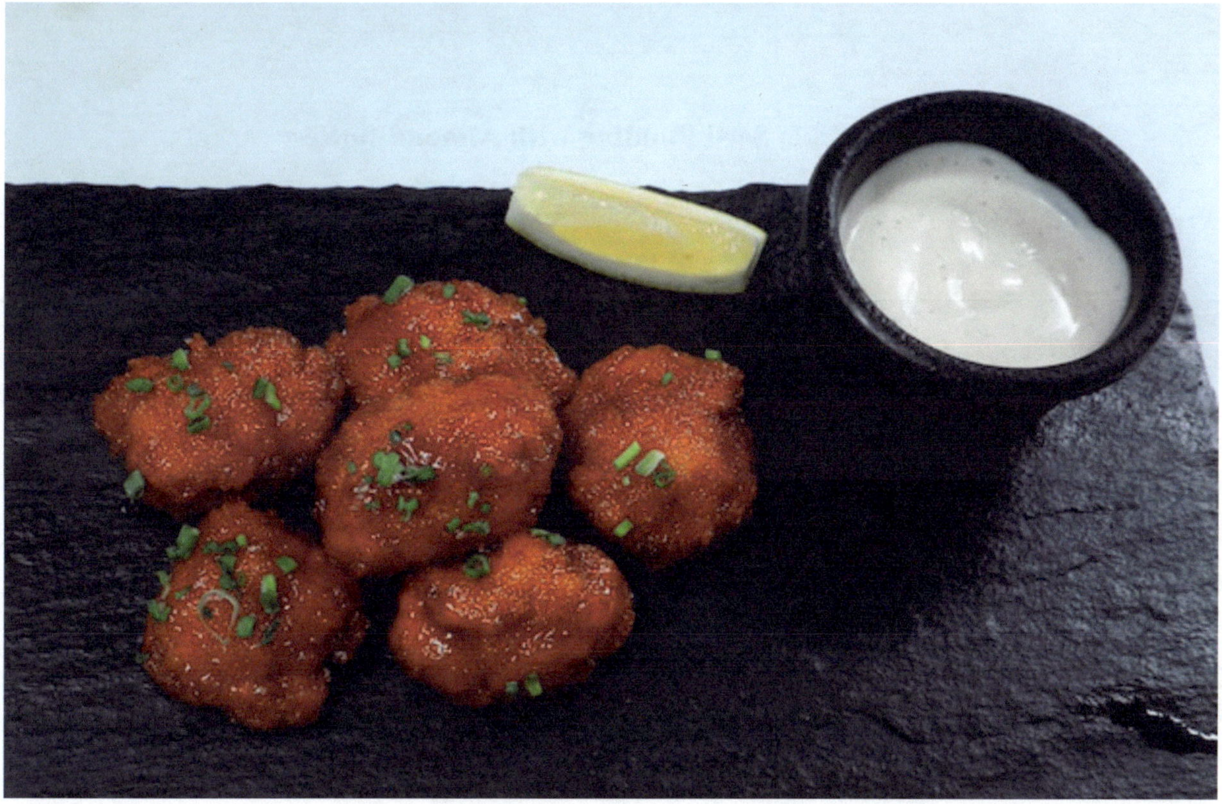

85. Cauliflower Bites with Buffalo Sauce

Prep.Time: 10 min

Cook Time: 20-25 min

Serving: 1

Beverage pairing: Lemonade

Ingredients:

- 2 cups cauliflower florets
- 2 tablespoons olive oil
- Salt and pepper to taste
- Buffalo sauce (sugar-free)

Preparation:

1. Preheat the oven to 425°F (220°C).
2. In a bowl, toss cauliflower florets with olive oil until evenly coated.
3. Season with salt and pepper to taste.
4. Spread the cauliflower florets on a baking sheet lined with parchment paper.
5. Roast in the preheated oven for 20-25 minutes, until golden brown and tender.
6. Drizzle with buffalo sauce before serving.

Nutrient Facts (per serving):

- Calories: Approximately 100 per serving
- Carbohydrates: 8g
- Fat: 7g
- Protein: 3g

86. Chia Seed Pudding with Almond Butter

Prep.Time: 5 min	Cook Time: 0 min	Serving: 1	Beverage pairing: Water

Ingredients:

- 1/4 cup chia seeds
- 1 cup unsweetened almond milk
- 1 tablespoon almond butter
- Optional: Sweetener of choice (such as honey or maple syrup)

Preparation:

1. In a bowl or jar, mix together chia seeds and almond milk.
2. Stir in almond butter until well combined.
3. Optional: Sweeten with honey or maple syrup to taste.
4. Cover and refrigerate for at least 2 hours, or overnight, until thickened.
5. Serve chilled with a dollop of almond butter on top.

Nutrient Facts (per serving):

- Calories: Approximately 200 per serving
- Carbohydrates: 15g
- Fat: 12g
- Protein: 8g

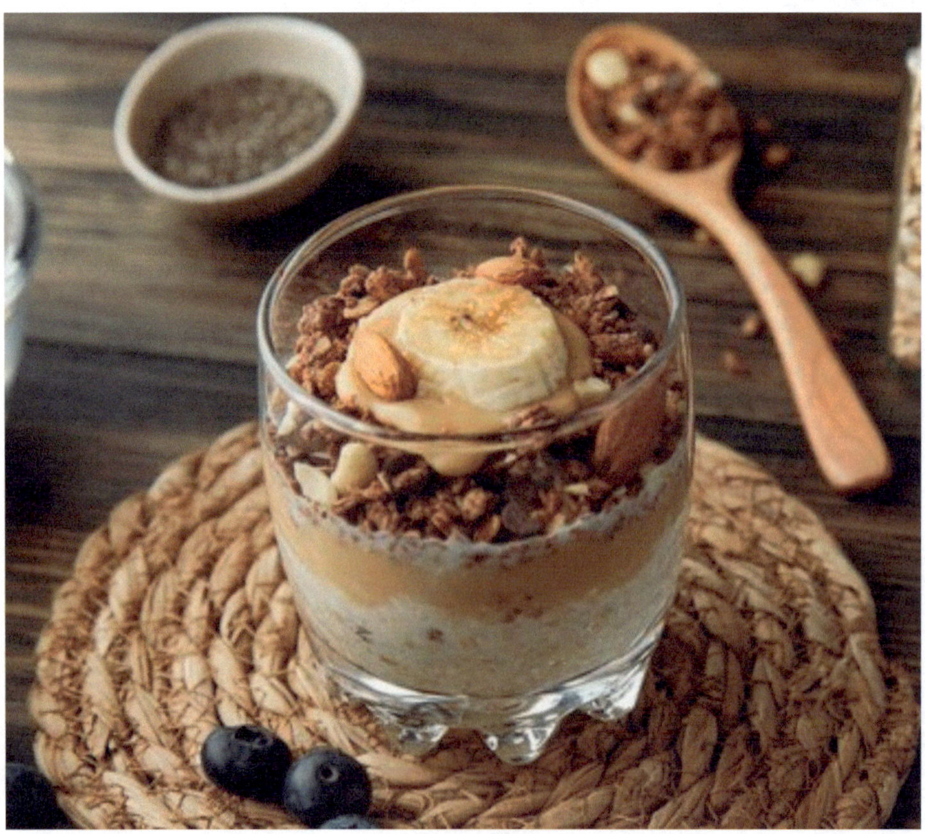

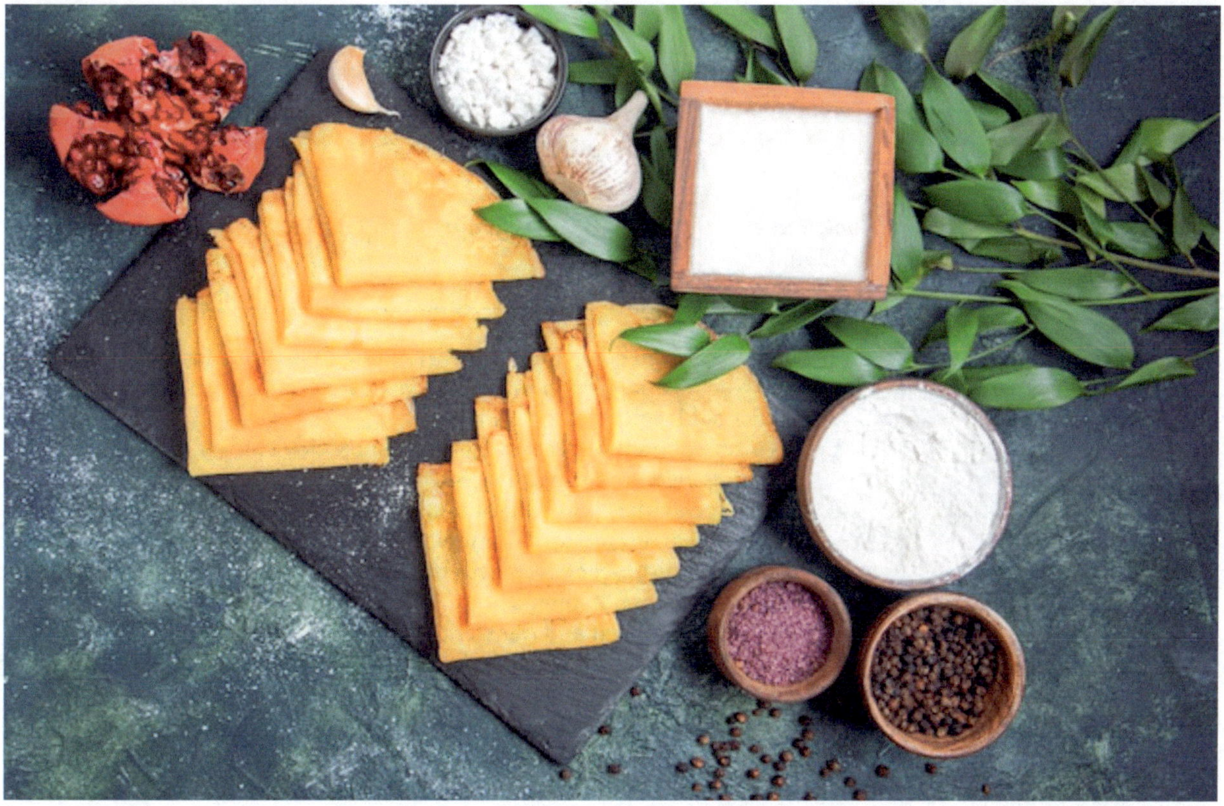

87. Baked Cheese Crisps with Rosemary

Prep.Time: 5 min | **Cook Time:** 5-7 min | **Serving:** 1 | **Beverage pairing:** Black Coffee

Ingredients:

- 1 cup shredded cheese (such as cheddar or Parmesan)
- 1 teaspoon chopped fresh rosemary

Preparation:

1. Preheat the oven to 350°F (175°C). Line a baking sheet with parchment paper.
2. Arrange small piles of shredded cheese on the prepared baking sheet, leaving space between each pile.
3. Sprinkle chopped fresh rosemary over each pile of cheese.
4. Bake in the preheated oven for 5-7 minutes, or until the edges are golden and crisp.
5. Let cool before serving.

Nutrient Facts (per serving):

- Calories: Approximately 100 per serving
- Carbohydrates: 1g
- Fat: 8g
- Protein: 6g

89. Soy-Ginger Edamame

Prep.Time:	Cook Time:	Serving:	Beverage pairing:
15 min	5-7 min	1	Green Tea

Ingredients:

- 2 cups edamame (fresh or frozen)
- 2 tablespoons soy sauce (low-sodium if preferred)
- 1 tablespoon rice vinegar
- 1 tablespoon honey or maple syrup
- 1 teaspoon grated fresh ginger
- 1 clove garlic, minced
- 1 teaspoon sesame seeds (optional)
- Pinch of red pepper flakes (optional)
- Fresh cilantro leaves for garnish (optional)

Preparation:

1. If using frozen edamame, cook according to package instructions. If using fresh edamame, blanch in boiling water for 5 minutes, then drain and rinse under cold water.
2. In a small bowl, whisk together soy sauce, rice vinegar, honey or maple syrup, grated ginger, and minced garlic to make the sauce.
3. In a large skillet, heat a bit of oil over medium heat. Add the cooked edamame and sauté for 2-3 minutes.
4. Pour the soy-ginger sauce over the edamame and toss to coat evenly. Cook for an additional 2 minutes.
5. Remove from heat and transfer the edamame to a serving dish.
6. Sprinkle sesame seeds and red pepper flakes over the edamame if desired.
7. Garnish with fresh cilantro leaves.
8. Serve hot or at room temperature as a delicious and nutritious snack.

Nutrient Facts (per serving):

- Calories: Approximately 120 per serving (1/2 cup)
- Carbohydrates: 9g
- Fat: 5g
- Protein: 11g

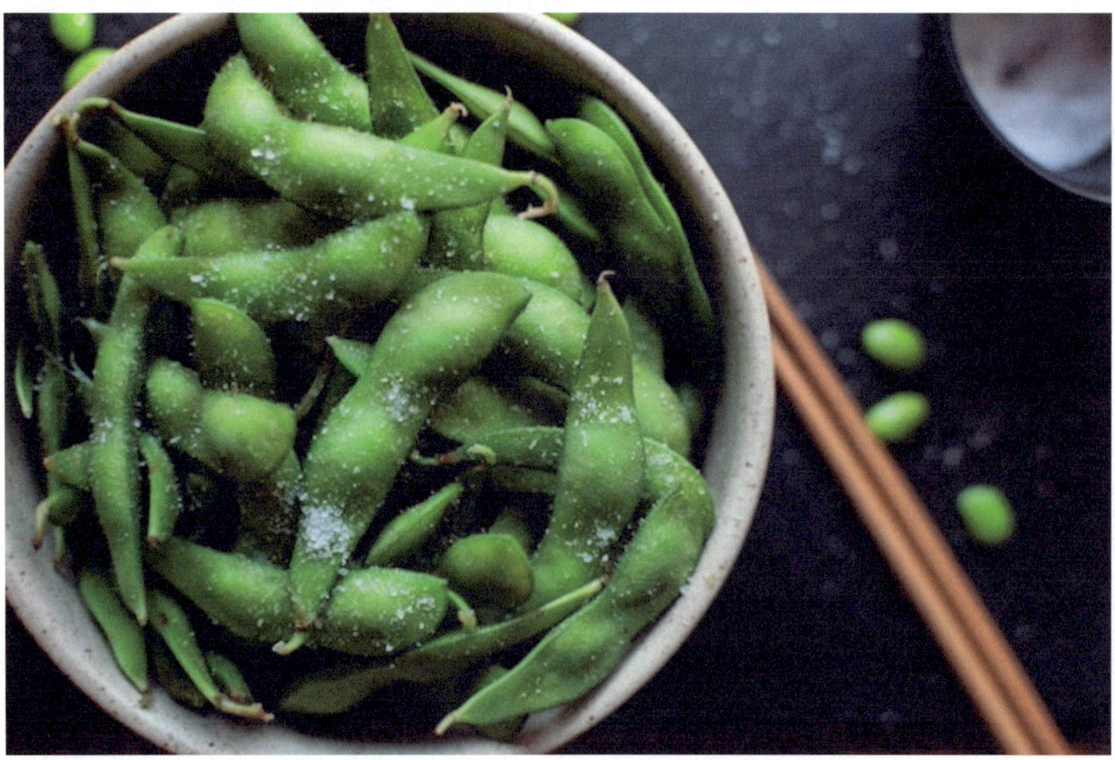

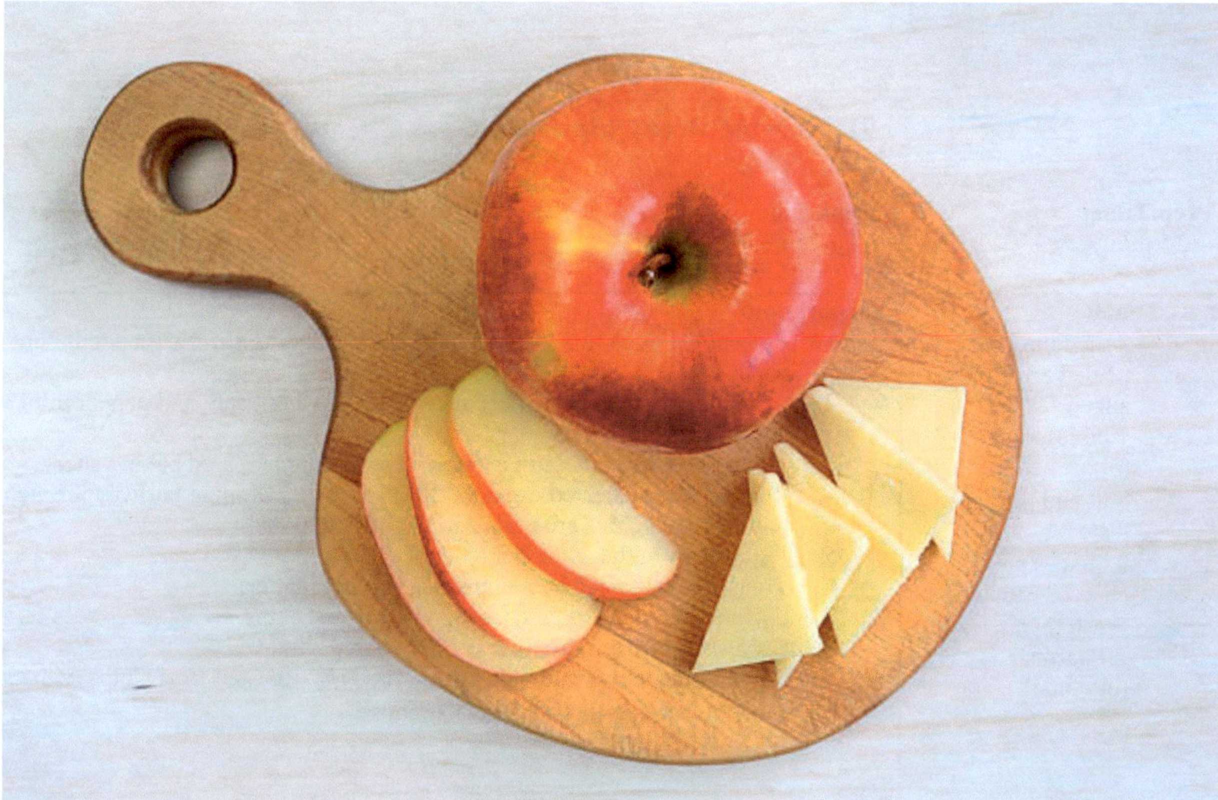

90. Cheddar Cheese and Apple Stacks

Prep.Time: 5 min

Cook Time: 5 min

Serving: 1

Beverage pairing: Cranberry Juice

Ingredients:

- 1 apple, cored and sliced into rounds
- 2 slices cheddar cheese
- 1 tablespoon honey or maple syrup (optional)
- 1 tablespoon chopped walnuts or pecans (optional)

Preparation:

1. Place a slice of cheddar cheese on top of each apple round.
2. Drizzle honey or maple syrup over the cheese if desired.
3. Sprinkle chopped walnuts or pecans on top if desired.
4. Stack another apple round on top to make a "sandwich."
5. Repeat with the remaining apple slices and cheese.
6. Serve immediately and enjoy these delicious and satisfying Cheddar Cheese and Apple Stacks as a quick and easy snack.

Nutrient Facts (per serving):

- Calories: Approximately 150 per serving (1 stack)
- Carbohydrates: 10g
- Fat: 10g
- Protein: 7g

91. Roasted Beet Chips with Goat Cheese

Prep.Time:	Cook Time:	Serving:	Beverage pairing:
15 min	20-25 min	1	Almond Milk

Ingredients:

- 2 medium beets, peeled and thinly sliced
- 1 tablespoon olive oil
- Salt and pepper to taste
- 2 ounces goat cheese, crumbled
- Fresh thyme leaves for garnish (optional)

Preparation:

1. Preheat the oven to 375°F (190°C). Line a baking sheet with parchment paper.
2. In a large bowl, toss the beet slices with olive oil, salt, and pepper until evenly coated.
3. Arrange the beet slices in a single layer on the prepared baking sheet.
4. Roast in the preheated oven for 20-25 minutes, flipping halfway through, until the beet chips are crisp and slightly browned.
5. Remove from the oven and let cool slightly.
6. Transfer the roasted beet chips to a serving platter.
7. Sprinkle crumbled goat cheese over the beet chips.
8. Garnish with fresh thyme leaves if desired.
9. Serve immediately and enjoy these flavorful Roasted Beet Chips with Goat Cheese as a delicious and healthy snack.

Nutrient Facts (per serving):

- Calories: Approximately 130 per serving (1/2 cup)
- Carbohydrates: 10g
- Fat: 7g
- Protein: 4g

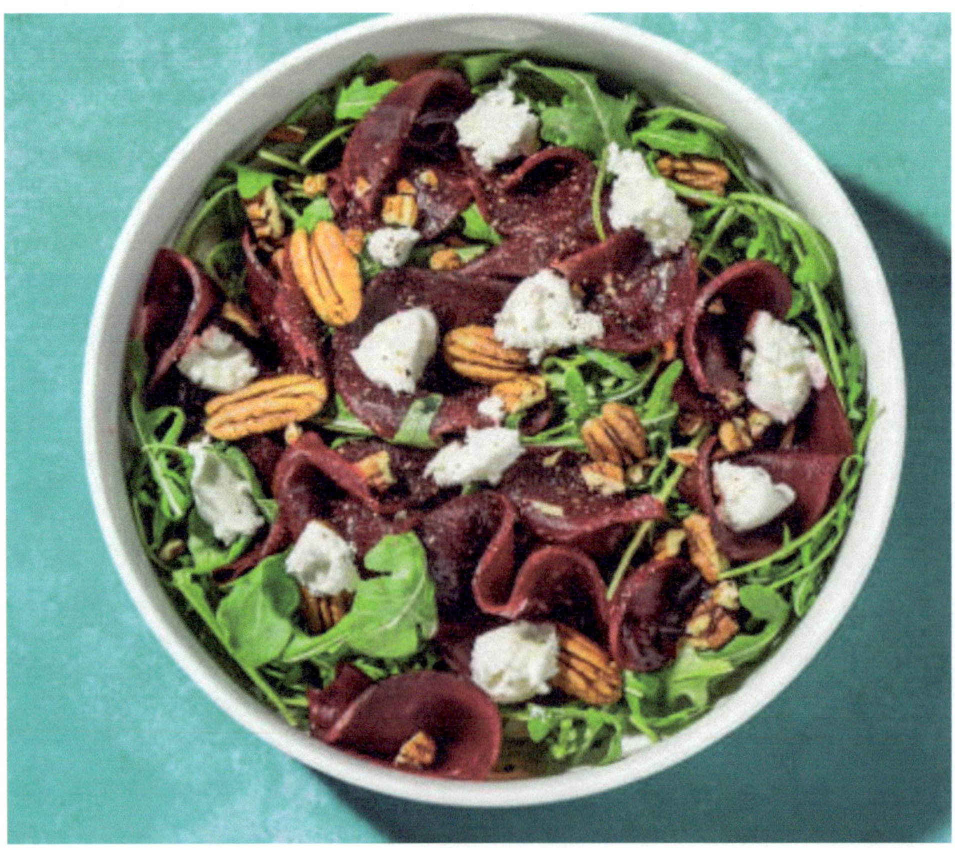

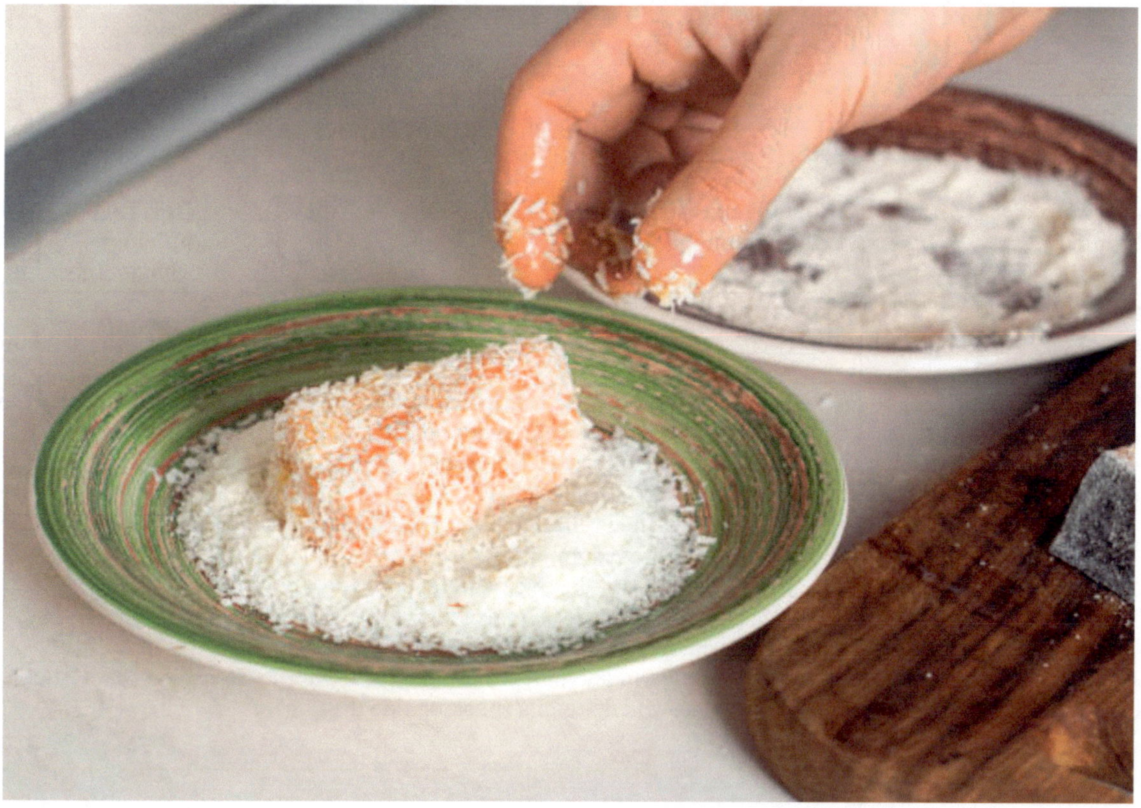

92. Coconut-Crusted Tofu Bites

Prep.Time: 20 min | **Cook Time:** 10 min | **Serving:** 1 | **Beverage pairing:** Lemonade

Ingredients:

- 1 block firm tofu, pressed and cut into bite-sized cubes
- 1/4 cup unsweetened shredded coconut
- 1/4 cup almond flour
- 1 teaspoon garlic powder
- 1/2 teaspoon paprika
- Salt and pepper to taste
- 1 egg, beaten (or alternative milk for vegan option)
- Coconut oil for frying

Preparation:

1. In a shallow dish, mix together shredded coconut, almond flour, garlic powder, paprika, salt, and pepper.
2. Dip each tofu cube into the beaten egg (or alternative milk), then coat evenly with the coconut mixture.
3. Heat coconut oil in a skillet over medium heat.
4. Fry the coconut-crusted tofu cubes in the hot oil until golden brown and crispy on all sides, about 2-3 minutes per side.
5. Remove from the skillet and place on a plate lined with paper towels to drain excess oil.
6. Serve immediately with your favorite dipping sauce, such as sweet chili sauce or soy sauce.
7. Enjoy these flavorful and crispy Coconut-Crusted Tofu Bites as a delicious and satisfying snack or appetizer.

Nutrient Facts (per serving):

- Calories: Approximately 180 per serving (4 pieces)
- Carbohydrates: 9g
- Fat: 12g
- Protein: 10g

93. Paprika Roasted Carrot Sticks

Prep.Time: 10 min

Cook Time: 20-25 min

Serving: 1

Beverage pairing: Ginger Tea

Ingredients:

- 4 large carrots, peeled and cut into sticks
- 1 tablespoon olive oil
- 1 teaspoon paprika
- 1/2 teaspoon garlic powder
- Salt and pepper to taste
- Fresh parsley for garnish (optional)

Preparation:

1. Preheat the oven to 400°F (200°C). Line a baking sheet with parchment paper.
2. In a large bowl, toss the carrot sticks with olive oil, paprika, garlic powder, salt, and pepper until evenly coated.
3. Arrange the seasoned carrot sticks in a single layer on the prepared baking sheet.
4. Roast in the preheated oven for 20-25 minutes, or until the carrots are tender and slightly caramelized.
5. Remove from the oven and let cool slightly.
6. Transfer the roasted carrot sticks to a serving platter.
7. Garnish with fresh parsley if desired.
8. Serve warm and enjoy these flavorful Paprika Roasted Carrot Sticks as a healthy and delicious snack or side dish.

Nutrient Facts (per serving):

- Calories: Approximately 80 per serving (1/2 cup)
- Carbohydrates: 10g
- Fat: 4g
- Protein: 1g

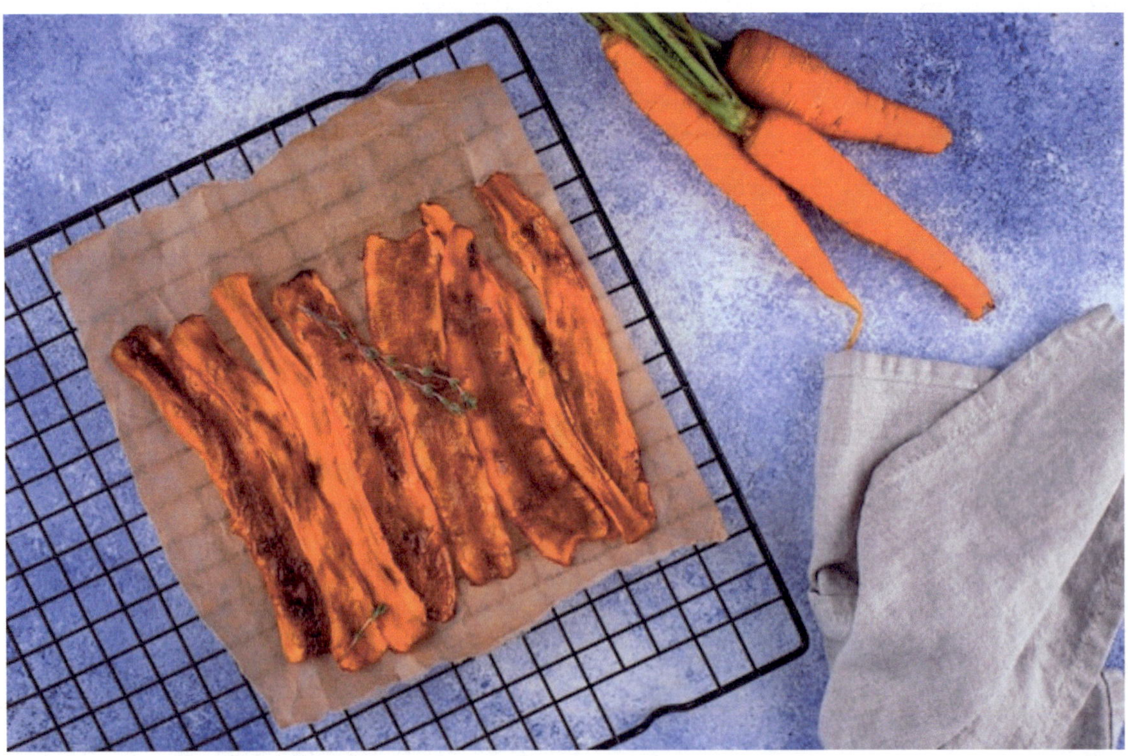

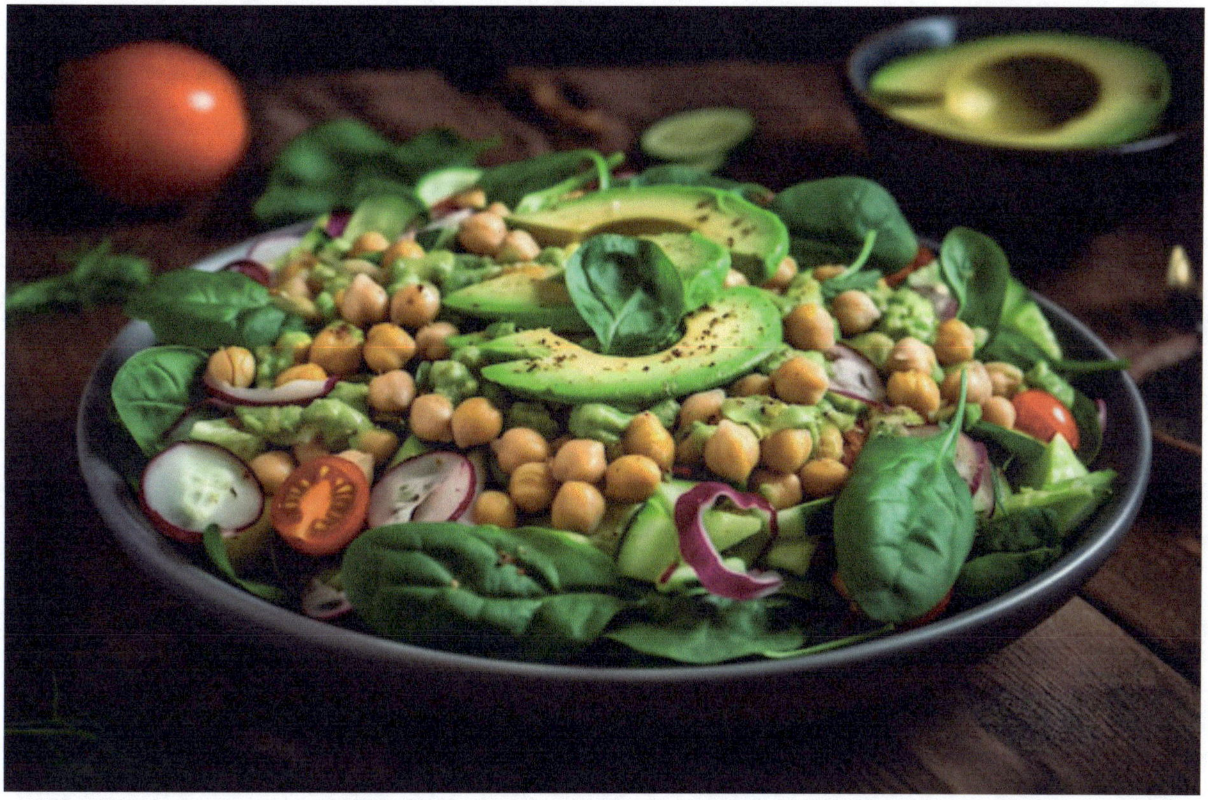

94. Spiced Chickpea and Spinach Salad

Prep.Time: 10 min

Cook Time: 20-25 min

Serving: 1

Beverage pairing: Cucumber Water

Ingredients:

- 1 can (15 ounces) chickpeas, drained and rinsed
- 1 tablespoon olive oil
- 1 teaspoon ground cumin
- 1/2 teaspoon smoked paprika
- Salt and pepper to taste
- 4 cups fresh spinach leaves
- 1/4 cup sliced red onion
- 1/4 cup crumbled feta cheese (optional)
- 1 tablespoon balsamic vinegar
- 1 tablespoon lemon juice

Preparation:

1. Preheat the oven to 400°F (200°C). Line a baking sheet with parchment paper.
2. In a bowl, toss the chickpeas with olive oil, ground cumin, smoked paprika, salt, and pepper until evenly coated.
3. Spread the seasoned chickpeas in a single layer on the prepared baking sheet. Roast in the preheated oven for 20-25 minutes, stirring halfway through, until the chickpeas are crispy.
4. In a large bowl, combine the roasted chickpeas, fresh spinach leaves, sliced red onion, and crumbled feta cheese (if using).
5. Drizzle balsamic vinegar and lemon juice over the salad.
6. Toss gently to combine.
7. Serve immediately and enjoy this flavorful and nutritious Spiced Chickpea and Spinach Salad as a light and satisfying snack or side dish.

Nutrient Facts (per serving):

- Calories: Approximately 180 per serving (1 cup)
- Carbohydrates: 25g
- Fat: 7g
- Protein: 8g

95. Cheese and Olive Skewers

Prep.Time:	Cook Time:	Serving:	Beverage pairing:
5 min	0 min	1	Mint Tea

Ingredients:

- Cubes of cheese (such as cheddar, mozzarella, or feta)
- Pitted olives (green or black)

Preparation:

1. Thread cubes of cheese and pitted olives onto skewers.
2. Serve as a simple and flavorful snack or appetizer.

Nutrient Facts (per serving):

- Calories: Approximately 150 per serving
- Carbohydrates: 2g
- Fat: 12g
- Protein: 8g

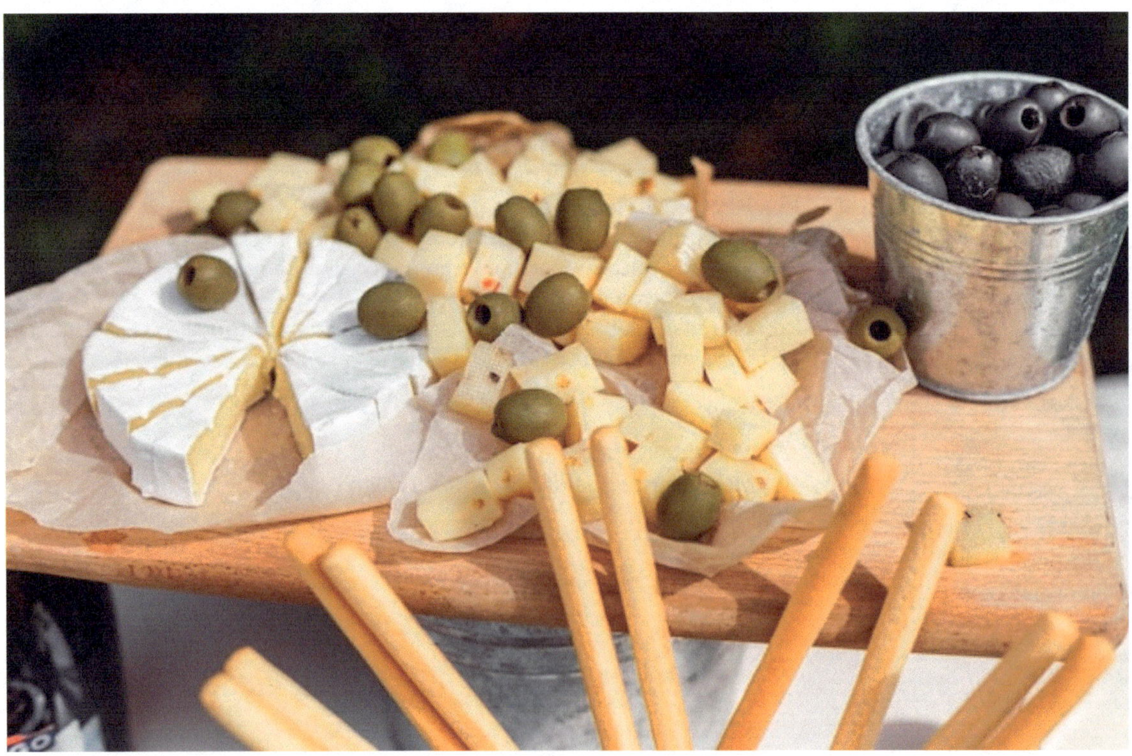

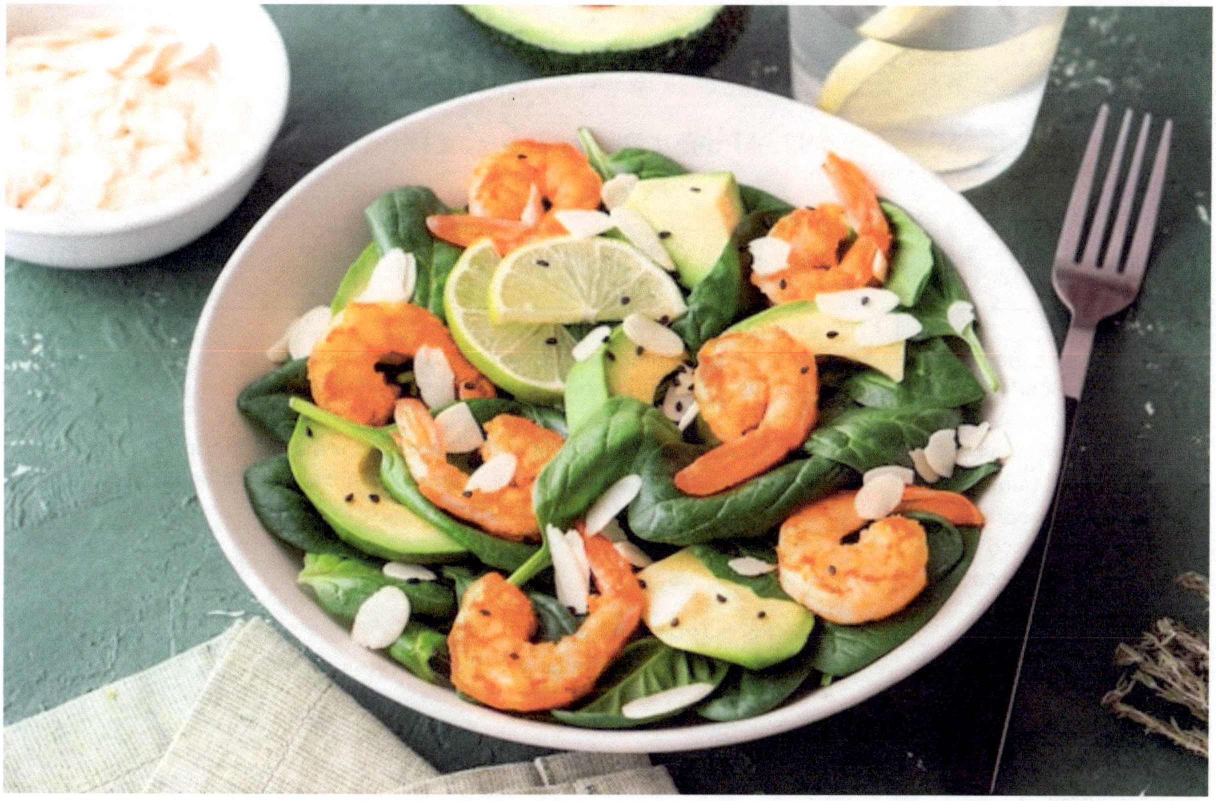

96. Avocado and Shrimp Salad

Prep.Time: 5 min

Cook Time: 5 min

Serving: 1

Beverage pairing: Herbal Tea

Ingredients:

- 1 ripe avocado, diced
- Cooked shrimp, peeled and deveined
- Mixed salad greens
- Dressing of choice (sugar-free)

Preparation:

1. In a bowl, combine diced avocado, cooked shrimp, and mixed salad greens.
2. Drizzle with dressing of choice and toss until well combined.
3. Serve immediately as a light and satisfying salad.

Nutrient Facts (per serving):

- Calories: Approximately 200 per serving
- Carbohydrates: 5g
- Fat: 12g
- Protein: 18g

97. Almond Butter Banana Bites

Prep.Time:	Cook Time:	Serving:	Beverage pairing:
5 min	0 min	1	Cinnamon Tea

Ingredients:

- 1 large banana, peeled and sliced into rounds
- 2 tablespoons almond butter
- 2 tablespoons unsweetened shredded coconut (optional)
- 2 tablespoons chopped almonds (optional)
- 1 tablespoon honey or maple syrup (optional)

Preparation:

1. Spread almond butter on top of each banana round.
2. If using, sprinkle shredded coconut and chopped almonds over the almond butter.
3. Drizzle honey or maple syrup over the toppings if desired.
4. Serve immediately and enjoy these simple and delicious Almond Butter Banana Bites as a nutritious snack or dessert.

Nutrient Facts (per serving):

- Calories: Approximately 120 per serving (2 bites)
- Carbohydrates: 15g
- Fat: 6g
- Protein: 3g

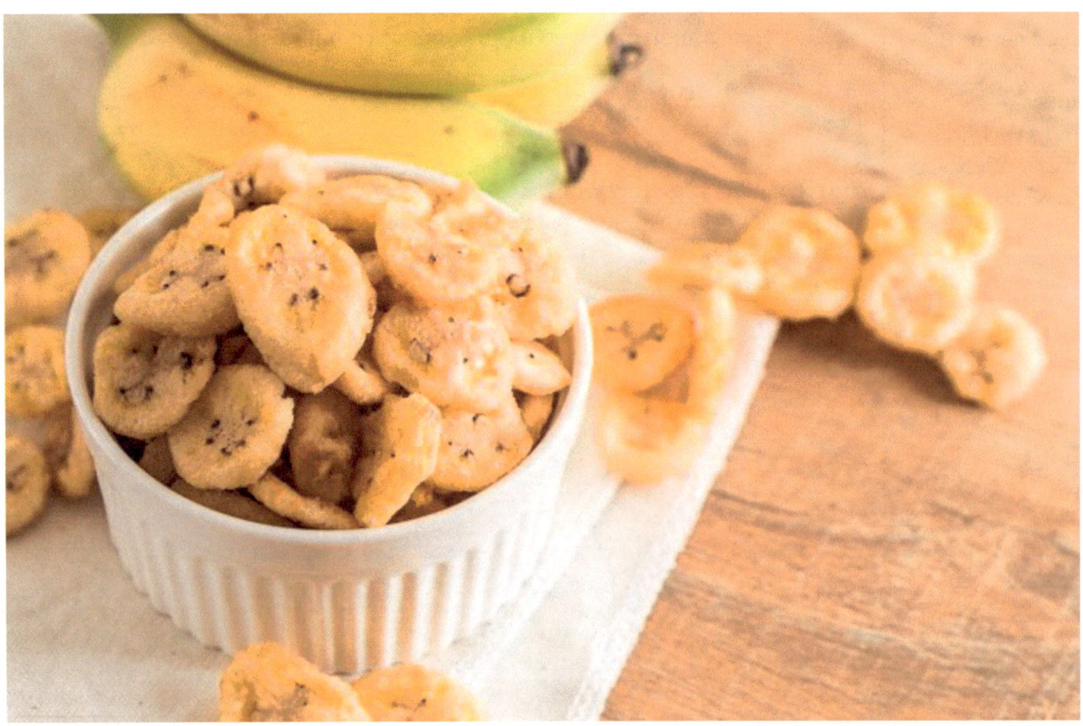

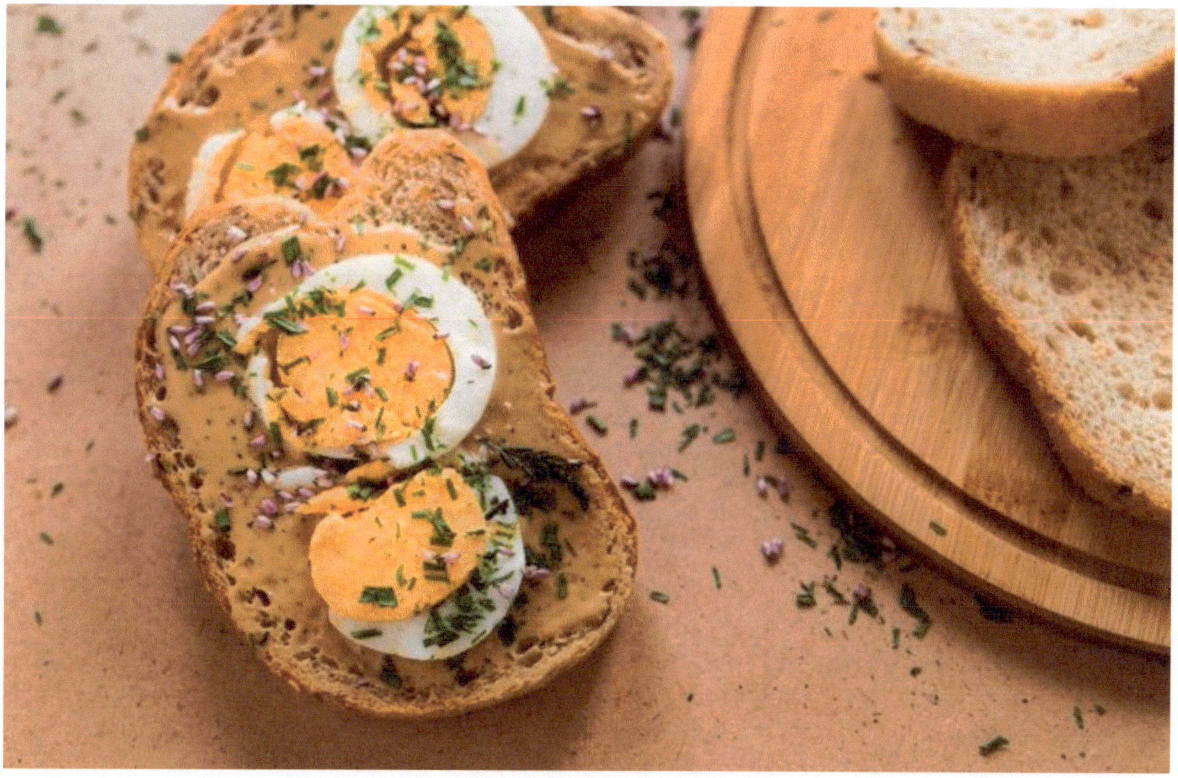

98. Hard-Boiled Eggs with Everything Bagel Seasoning

Prep.Time: 5 min	**Cook Time:** 10 min	**Serving:** 1	**Beverage pairing:** Black Coffee

Ingredients:

- Hard-boiled eggs
- Everything bagel seasoning

Preparation:

1. Peel hard-boiled eggs and slice in half lengthwise.
2. Sprinkle everything bagel seasoning over the egg halves.
3. Serve as a protein-rich snack or appetizer.

Nutrient Facts (per serving):

- Calories: Approximately 150 per serving
- Carbohydrates: 2g
- Fat: 10g
- Protein: 12g

99. Berry and Spinach Smoothie Bowl

Prep.Time:	Cook Time:	Serving:	Beverage pairing:
5 min	0 min	1	Water

Ingredients:

- 1 cup fresh spinach leaves
- 1/2 cup mixed berries (such as strawberries, blueberries, raspberries)
- 1/2 banana, frozen
- 1/2 cup unsweetened almond milk or coconut milk
- Toppings of choice (such as sliced banana, berries, nuts, seeds)

Preparation:

1. In a blender, combine fresh spinach leaves, mixed berries, frozen banana, and almond milk.
2. Blend until smooth and creamy, adding more liquid if necessary to reach desired consistency.
3. Pour the smoothie into a bowl.
4. Top with sliced banana, additional berries, nuts, seeds, or other toppings of choice.
5. Serve immediately with a spoon.

Nutrient Facts (per serving):

- Calories: Approximately 150 per serving
- Carbohydrates: 20g
- Fat: 5g
- Protein: 8g

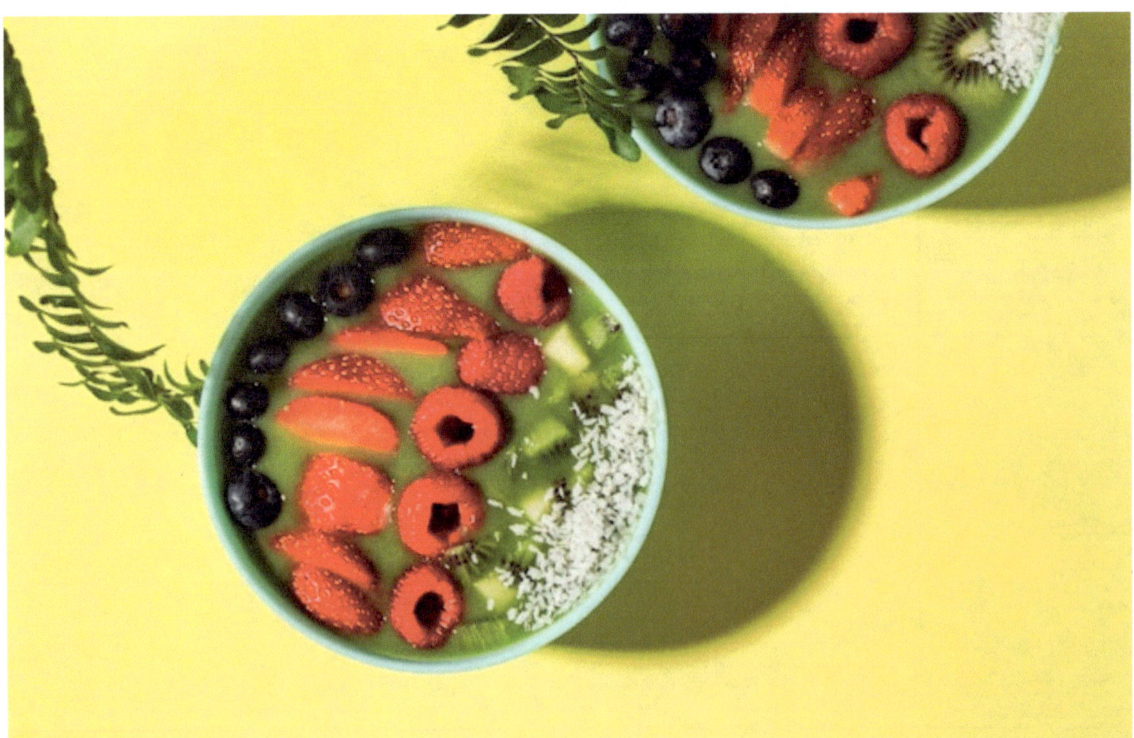

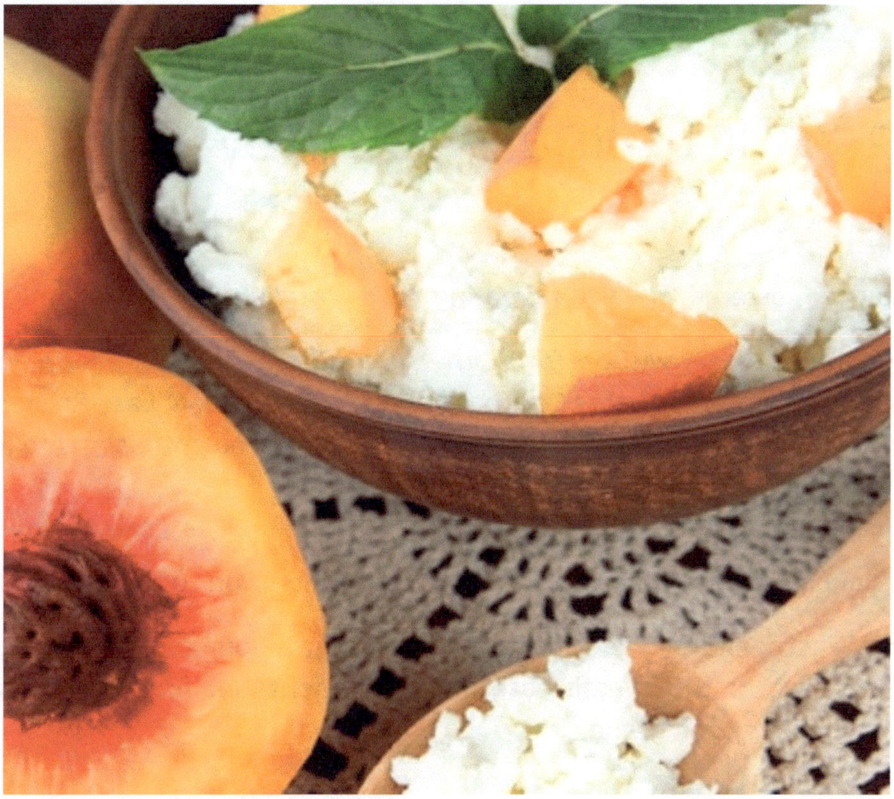

100. Cottage Cheese and Peach Slices

Prep.Time: 2 min

Cook Time: 0 min

Serving: 1

Beverage pairing: Herbal Tea

Ingredients:

- 1/2 cup cottage cheese
- 1 ripe peach, sliced

Preparation:

1. Place cottage cheese in a bowl.
2. Top with sliced peach.
3. Serve immediately and enjoy this simple and nutritious Cottage Cheese and Peach Slices as a refreshing snack or light meal.

Nutrient Facts (per serving):

- Calories: Approximately 120 per serving (1/2 cup cottage cheese with 1 peach)
- Carbohydrates: 15g
- Fat: 2g
- Protein: 12g

Sharing Your Culinary Journey

Now that you've mastered the art of creating delicious, diabetes-friendly meals, it's time to share your newfound culinary wisdom with others who are on the same path. By leaving your honest review of the "Type 2 Diabetes Cookbook: Beginner's Quick & Easy Recipes for Delicious Diabetes Diets" by Lily Anders on Amazon, you'll guide fellow food enthusiasts to a resource that can transform their dining table and health.

Your insights and experiences are invaluable, offering a beacon to those navigating their diet amidst diabetes. Whether it was a specific recipe that became your go-to, a tip that changed how you approach cooking, or the overall ease and enjoyment you found in these pages, your feedback is a gift that keeps on giving.

Thank you for contributing to a community of knowledge and support. The journey towards healthy eating and diabetes management thrives on shared discoveries and successes. By passing on your review, you're not just recommending a book—you're enriching lives with the joy of cooking and the empowerment of dietary control.

To leave your review, just follow this link:

https://www.amazon.com/review/create-review/?ie=UTF8&channel=glance-detail&asin=1963939360

Together, we're keeping the passion for healthy, joyful eating alive, one review at a time. Your support makes all the difference, not just to us, but to every reader and cook who seeks to balance their love for food with their health needs.

- With heartfelt thanks,

Lily Anders

Conclusion

In conclusion, this book transcends the traditional approach to managing diabetes through diet alone, offering a comprehensive guide that empowers individuals with diabetes to navigate their condition with knowledge and precision. Through 300 carefully crafted recipes, we explore the importance of balancing nutrient intake and the vital role of consistent meal planning. Each recipe is not just a set of instructions but a building block towards a healthier life, tailored to the unique needs of those managing diabetes.

As we close this journey of understanding and adaptation, remember that managing diabetes is not just about adhering to dietary restrictions or grappling with numbers—it is about reclaiming control of your health and life. These recipes are designed not only to meet specific nutritional needs but also to delight the palate, proving that a diabetes-conscious diet can be as delicious as it is nutritious.

Embrace these culinary tools as your allies in the pursuit of wellness. Let each meal enrich your body and spirit, and may the knowledge contained in this book guide you toward a balanced, joyful, and healthy life with diabetes. Here's to finding pleasure in every bite and strength in every challenge. Cheers to your health and happiness on this flavorful journey!

Made in the USA
Monee, IL
14 September 2026

62980075R00072

SNACKS

Snacking is often where Type 2 Diabetes feels most challenging. Hunger strikes between meals, and choices can feel limited or risky.

TYPE 2 DIABETES COOKBOOK: SNACKS OFFERS SIMPLE, BALANCED SOLUTIONS.

This book features diabetes-friendly snacks designed to curb hunger, stabilize blood sugar, and support consistency throughout the day.

Each option is practical, portion-aware, and easy to enjoy without guilt.

SNACKS SHOULD SUPPORT YOUR DAY,

NOT COMPLICATE IT.

ISBN 9781963939842

90000

9 781963 939842